The Battle for the High Street

Phil Hubbard

The Battle for the High Street

Retail Gentrification, Class and Disgust

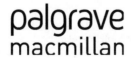

Phil Hubbard
King's College London
Department of Geography
London, UK

ISBN 978-1-137-52152-1   ISBN 978-1-137-52153-8   (eBook)
DOI 10.1057/978-1-137-52153-8

Library of Congress Control Number: 2016947442

Cover image © Mark Wiener / Alamy Stock Photo

Printed on acid-free paper

This Palgrave Macmillan imprint is published by Springer Nature
The registered company is Macmillan Publishers Ltd.
The registered company address is: The Campus, 4 Crinan Street, London, N1 9XW, United Kingdom

Acknowledgements

This book is one that has been intimately shaped by my personal circumstances, and in particular, returning to the county of my birth some quarter of a century after leaving. In that time, much had changed in the local towns and villages, including in some cases a rapid gentrification that had changed these places beyond recognition. Reflecting on some of these changes, and discussing these with my work colleagues, spurred me to write this book, which in many ways is my attempt to show how the sociological preoccupation with class (and the language of class) remains relevant to urban theory, notwithstanding the popularity of alternative ways of reading the urban landscape. In this sense, I am particularly thankful to those colleagues at the University of Kent who indulged me over the last five years as I have suggested ways in which the reconfiguration of Whitstable and Margate (and some of the other places that feature prominently in this book) illustrate wider transitions in the nature of post-industrial culture. Here, I should particularly mention Anne Bottomley, David Garbin, Ben Hickman, Dawn Lyon, Vince Miller, David Nettleingham, and Tim Strangleman, as well as acknowledging the support of the School of Social Policy, Sociology and Social Research, which provided a stimulating inter-disciplinary environment. I have also benefitted from discussions with graduate students, especially Jon Ward, whose work on artistic labour in seaside towns significantly informed the writing of Chap. 9, and Deanna Dadusc, whose research on urban social movements and squatting has challenged me to think about questions of resistance in an era when gentrification often seems the 'only game in town'. Beyond Kent, I owe a debt of thanks to those who looked at this book in part or whole and suggested changes (inevitably, not all of which I was able to accommodate): these include Nick Clarke, Louise Crewe, Suzanne Hall, Brian Hracs, Mark Jayne, Loretta Lees, and Neil Wrigley. I am also grateful to the Departments of Geography at Malmo, Birmingham and the LSE where I presented versions of these chapters, as well as the different public audiences I have presented this research to in Margate. This said, some of the arguments in this book have had a much longer gestation and have benefitted from varied intellectual inputs from colleagues and friends over two decades. For example, some of the material on disadvantaged consumers presented here is informed by the work I conducted with colleagues at Coventry University in the 1990s, and here I should particularly mention Nigel Berkeley, Phil Dunham and Peter Williams. Likewise, material on nightlife and the 24-hour city was presented and discussed with numerous colleagues at Loughborough University with a Nuffield-funded project on cinema-going helping focus my thinking on the move 'out of town' as discussed in Chap. 3. The arguments presented in Chap. 6 are in part derived from a study undertaken with Rachela Colosi supported by Economic and Social Research Council grant ES/J002755/1 'Sexualisation, nuisance and safety: sexual entertainment venues and the management of risk'. Here, thanks are owing to Rachela Colosi and the Research Associate on that project, Billie Lister. Finally, I owe a massive debt of gratitude to Eleanor for her close and critical reading of the manuscript, as well as her constant support during the twelve months it took to complete it.

Contents

List of Figures

1

Introduction: Gentrification and Retail Change

The literature on contemporary cities is vast, constantly evolving as it struggles to keep pace with frenetic processes of urban restructuring. But for the last 50 years or so, one theoretical concept has consistently been to the fore: urban gentrification. Originally invoked to describe the social transformation of some of London's inner city neighbourhoods via the 'sweat equity' of owner-occupiers, the term is now routinely used to describe any instance where landscapes of long-term disinvestment are 'upscaled' through state funding, corporate speculation or individual initiative. Around the world, we are seeing neighbourhoods long associated with working-class and minority populations being reinvented in accordance with contemporary ideals of metropolitan living, with new residents and tourists consuming these spaces as sites of leisured, middle-class urbanity. Corporations search eagerly for new opportunities to exploit the 'rent gap' between current and potential rents, often aided and abetted by state governors keen to see an urban transformation. The theories and experiences of gentrification first worked through in London in the 1960s are thus being updated and revised as new landscapes and spaces of gentrification become apparent elsewhere, including the global South. Indeed, the putative globalization of gentrification has led some

© The Editor(s) (if applicable) and The Author(s) 2017
P. Hubbard, *The Battle for the High Street*,
DOI 10.1057/978-1-137-52153-8_1

scholars to suggest the pulse behind gentrification is now generalized, and a key dimension of 'planetary urbanism' (Merrifield 2013; Wyly 2015).

But gentrification is not just diffusing globally, with the gentrification 'frontier' simultaneously moving out from the inner city to encompass other locations. Affluent, cosmopolitan groups are colonizing outer as well as inner suburbs, villages as well as urban neighbourhoods, provincial towns as well as world cities. Many new inflections and varieties of gentrification have been delimited: black gentrification, super-gentrification, gay gentrification, touristification, greentrification, studentification and so forth (Lauria and Knopp 1985; Butler and Lees 2006; Gotham 2005; Smith and Holt 2007; Moore 2009). All demonstrate that specific middle-class identities can become valued in processes of development and regeneration and stress the locally diverse forms gentrification takes as it becomes a global urban strategy (Smith 2002). All contribute to our understanding of the processes of uneven development that are part and parcel of our urbanized existence and stress that gentrification is not always imitative, involving the intersection of generalized and local processes that existing theorizations do not always fully capture (Lees 2012).

So the literature on gentrification has proliferated, expanding into new territories and producing novel understandings of the urban process. But despite this, some key battlegrounds of gentrification remain little studied. Shopping streets provide perhaps the best example. Despite the fact that the reinvention of local shopping streets as spaces of affluent, leisured consumption is a globally recognized phenomenon, and profoundly changing the character of some neighbourhoods, retail change remains poorly theorized as a form of gentrification. Indeed, in some overviews of gentrification (e.g. Lees et al. 2011), retailing has hardly been mentioned at all, with local shopping streets presumed to reflect the socio-economic character of surrounding neighbourhoods rather than in any sense driving the changes occurring in those spaces. So while it has been suggested local retail provides 'a particularly sensitive indicator of the balance of forces in gentrified neighbourhoods' (Bridge and Dowling 2001: 99), it's new-build, 'scorched-earth' gentrification, and the redevelopment of housing, that tends to preoccupy gentrification scholars, not the slow, sometimes subtle changes occurring on local shopping streets. As Katharine Rankin and Heather McLean (2015) assert, the consequence is that retail spaces have been imagined as essentially distinct from the residential spaces and neighbourhoods characterized as the leading edge of the gentrification frontier.

However, this epiphenomenal view of retail change is being challenged in the emerging, mainly North American, literature that's beginning to acknowledge the fundamental importance of retail change in instigating gentrification (e.g. Deener 2007; Sullivan 2014; Rankin and McLean 2015; Kern 2015a; Kasinitz and Zukin 2016). In these studies, the replacement of corner cafés by coffee shops, convenience grocery stores by delis and pubs by wine bars is depicted as a vital first stage in gentrification processes which culminate in the upscaling of entire neighbourhoods. New York-based cultural commentator Sharon Zukin and colleagues have provided one of the most influential accounts of these processes:

> At least since the 1970s, certain types of restaurants, cafés and stores have become highly visible signs of gentrification… Although the archetypal quiche-serving "fern bars" of the early years have long since yielded to wine bars and designer clothing boutiques, these stylish commercial spaces still embody, serve, and represent a powerful discourse of neighborhood change. On the most basic level, the new consumption spaces supply the material needs of more affluent residents and newcomers… But they also supply their less tangible needs for social and cultural capital… New stores, cafés and bars become hangouts for both bohemians and gentrifiers or places for social networking among stroller-pushing parents and underemployed artists and writers. (Zukin et al. 2009: 47)

Zukin et al. (2009) argue the economic and cultural entrepreneurs establishing new retail businesses in previously deprived districts (e.g. Williamsburg, Brooklyn) seek to fabricate an 'aura of authenticity' based on the working-class history of the area. In doing so, they initially capitalize on their reputation among a youthful, artistic clientele ('hipsters') seeking an authentic alternative to mainstream consumption space, attracting a broader middle-class consumer base over time. And, as Zukin et al. (2016) note, even modest injections of investment can bring a 'new look' to a shabby shopping street, with good write-ups in the local media and word-of-mouth publicity bringing more new investors: shoppers, diners, residents, real estate developers, and retail entrepreneurs. In time, rents rise, with the synergistic combination of retail and residential gentrification ultimately producing neighbourhoods associated with conspicuous consumption and middle-class rituals of belonging. Longer-term working-class residents are priced out of the neighbourhood, and cast culturally adrift.

Here, Zukin et al follow in the tradition of Michael Jager (1986), Caroline Mills (1988), David Ley (2003) and others who have focused on the consumption values of the gentrifying middle class when explaining the remaking of the central city. The argument here is well rehearsed. Middle-class gentrifiers, who lack the resources to copy upper-class consumer habits, rely on the revival and refurbishment of older, cheaper properties prized for their aesthetic potential, and they set about furnishing their house with similarly recycled vintage goods. This can even manifest in 'poor chic' (Halnon 2002), the process in which the middle classes seek to display distinction via the 'victorious' aesthetic consumption of lower-class symbolism. But poor chic does not involve the simple purchase of, and display of, second-hand or discount goods. It requires serious disposable income to clean and restore such goods, turning the merely shabby into 'shabby chic'. Working class authenticity is cherished, but in the process, it's symbolically consumed until little trace of its 'dirty' working-class background remains. Retail gentrification literatures suggest the same can be said of entire neighbourhoods, with 'sketchy' or marginal districts becoming 'crunchy' or 'hip' neighbourhoods before ultimately becoming internationally branded 'trendy' neighbourhoods by virtue of the arrival of designer stores and Michelin star restaurants (Kern 2015a).

A key idea in the retail gentrification literature is that the remaking of the retail landscape is central to the processes by which the inner city is served up as a *spectacle* to be consumed by the middle classes. Local shopping streets become not just spaces of economic and social reproduction, but spaces thoroughly integrated into circuits of middle-class display:

> Designer shops, art galleries, bars and restaurants form the background to a landscape of people in semi-public space (tables on the footpath they must pay to occupy) watching the passing parade and sipping chardonnay

from a boutique winery, beer from a microbrewery, coffee from organic beans grown in the developing country *du jour.* (Shaw 2008: 1698)

This colonization of space by conspicuous middle-class consumption suggests that the displacement of existing populations can occur through a range of different gentrification mechanisms. For example, whilst displacement is often thought to occur mainly via landlords raising rents, rendering housing unaffordable for existing residents (Newman and Wyly 2006), or through authorities instigating 'revanchist' policing strategies (Smith 1996), studies of retail gentrification show it can also occur through the indirect displacement instantiated by wholesale cultural changes at the local scale. Retail change is thought particularly significant in this respect: businesses change, pubs become wine bars, corner shops becomes delis, the greasy spoon café becomes a barista-style coffee shop and so on. Before long, the nature of the entire neighbourhood changes, and families and communities that may have been in place for years are broken up. As Peter Marcuse (1985: 207) asserts, 'when a family sees the neighbourhood around it changing dramatically, when their friends are leaving the neighbourhood, when the stores they patronise are liquidating and new stores for other clientele are taking their places ... then the pressure of displacement is severe'.

So while the improvement of shabby or part derelict shopping streets may be widely welcomed, it's clear retail change can drive long-term gentrification processes that are often far from benign. While advocates of regeneration agendas promoting the introduction of wealthier groups into middle-class communities defer (e.g. Freeman 2011), there's little evidence to back up claims that gentrification improves the conditions of the working-class residents who remain in gentrified communities. Indeed, most studies suggest displacement is a common outcome, with those displaced seldom settling successfully elsewhere (Goetz 2003; Kleit and Manzo 2006; Kearns and Mason 2013). So while retail gentrification can enhance the quality of local shopping provision, provide new economic opportunities and enhance the local built environment through re-aestheticization, the benefits are unequally felt. It's incomers who benefit from retail gentrification, with longer-term residents often forced to relocate where retail and cultural facilities are more in keeping with their tastes and budgets. The replacement of an 'ethnic' food store by a wholefood deli or upmarket boutique is not just a cultural transformation or 'whitening' of a local retail environment; it's also a class transformation that can be a harbinger of a more fundamental change in a locality.

This phenomenon—the transformation of local shopping streets into de facto spaces of gentrification—is now being explored in a variety of national contexts (see Zukin et al. 2016), with emerging evidence that this is being encouraged by state-led regeneration initiatives aiming to territorialize disinvested communities (McLean et al. 2015). But despite this, the concepts and language of retail gentrification are rarely deployed in Britain, with studies directly relating retail change to gentrification processes few and far between. A notable exception is Sara Gonzalez and Paul Waley's (2012) study of the redevelopment of a market in Leeds. Suggesting the authorities tend to see markets 'as mainly working-class spaces, cheap, unruly, wild, dirty, backwards', they argue that calls for markets to attract a wider range of urban residents—including 'the young, sleek suited, pin-striped city dwellers and professionals' (Gonzalez and Waley 2012: 7)—betrays a thoroughly classed language which imposes a symbolic violence on the less affluent. Their Leeds case study is echoed further north, with the closure of the traditional 'Paddy's Market', and the associated redevelopment of the Clyde waterfront and Merchant's City seen to underpin what Kirsteen Paton (2010) characterizes as the middle-class colonization of Glasgow. As she acerbically observes, 'the place is full of cafés for the café latte mob with their wee cakes' (Paton 2010: 219). Such studies figure marketplaces as one of the last bastions of working-class consumption in British towns and cities increasingly given over to leisured middle-class consumption (see also Dines 2009; Coles and Crang 2011). In this sense, they provide a valuable corrective to studies of 'new' forms of consumption (e.g. online retailing) by showing some populations remain reliant on more established retail channels. But more than this, they also highlight how retail change in Britain might be contributing to the exclusion of the working class from the spaces of the central city, a city increasingly given over to leisure, middle-class modes of consumption.

Appreciating that the upscaling of shopping districts in Britain creates exclusionary pressures is especially important in an area when local authorities and urban governors often seem to regard gentrification as the only game in town. One of the most blatant contradictions of our times is that 'neoliberal' urban policies justified as attempts to improve the conditions of the poor are predicated on making it as easy as possible for corporate developers to exploit the 'rent gap', with the working-class communities that provided the backbone of many cities' industrial economy being willingly sacrificed by urban politicians who seldom appear aware or concerned about the consequences of their actions. Too often the costs of gentrification for existing populations are ignored in accounts fixating on the material transformations associated with new development, some of which appear tacitly approving of the 'improvements' evident in given localities, whether this in the form of new housing, transport infrastructure or showy spaces of consumption. Shifting focus from studies of middle-class gentrifiers to the working class who bear the brunt of gentrification is then vital in a context where many academic studies of gentrification appear to be little more than 'performative instruments of public policy' effacing the relational geographies of class that characterize post-industrial cities (Davidson and Wyly 2012: 395).

It's this sense of injustice that has informed the writing of this book. Focusing on the British situation, its aim is to show that policies encouraging 'retail regeneration' are little concerned with recognizing the diverse needs of consumers, being fixated on certain middle-class modes of consumption and, in particular, the attraction of retro, hipster businesses including galleries, boutiques and 'real' coffee shops. Here, I seek to expose this pro-gentrification agenda via a critical reading of the many national policy documents and miscellaneous local initiatives launched over the last decade or so in the face of what is perceived to be a precipitous decline in the fortunes of the British High Street. Collectively, these map out an agenda for the revitalization of the High Street in which the case for retail regeneration, and the means by which this should be achieved, are left unquestioned. As will be described, far from recognizing the diverse ways that local shopping streets are produced and consumed, retail policies tend to suggest the fortunes of local shopping streets can only be revived by encouraging a particular brand of leisured consumption. 'Successful' High Streets are depicted as those that have cast off any taint of working-class consumption while failing ones are depicted as 'toxic', harbouring 'unhealthy' stores potentially off-putting to more affluent consumers and tourists.

In this book, I insist that the dominant policy vision of the High Street is inherently classed, with distinctions between 'failing' and 'thriving' shopping streets being informed by moralizing discourses distinguishing respectable from flawed forms of consumption. Adopting this critical perspective allows me to conceptualize retail policy in Britain as a form of moral regulation, an intervention promoting particular modes of consumption over others. My conclusion is that policies aiming to 'revive' British High Streets—for example, by replacing discount street markets with Farmers' Markets, pound-shops with niche boutiques and fast food takeaways with slow food vendors—might well succeed in transforming the fortunes of specific High Streets, but at a cost: the exclusion of the working-class populations who currently live, work and shop on and around these streets. This is by no means an original argument, as decades of urban scholarship and community sociology have suggested that regeneration often bequeaths gentrification. Time after time, we have witnessed incoming homeowners, economic entrepreneurs and property developers being the prime beneficiaries of measures ostensibly designed to improve the living and working environments of the poorest in society. Consider, for example, the impact of the 2012 London Olympics on house prices in the surrounding areas of Newham and Hackney (Kavetsos 2012). Here, rental increases since the Olympics of around £1200 a month on the average property have had a profoundly negative effect on young people seeking housing in the area, who are no longer able to live in the neighbourhoods where they grew up (witness the well-publicised campaign of the 'E15 mothers' to remain in their homes on the Carpenter's Estate in Stratford). A state-sponsored spectacular supposed to aid the poorest boroughs of London ended up supporting gentrification agendas, a repetition of one of the most familiar stories in contemporary urban studies. The middle classes take back the central city, assisted by 'neoliberal' urban policy, and the working class cast asunder.

Fighting against the pro-gentrification agendas implicit in British retail policy, a central tenet of this book is that contemporary British High Streets should not be described as dead or dying simply because they lack the stores and facilities idealized by middle-class consumer cultures. As I show, many 'failing' High Streets continue to play an important economic and social role in the lives of working-class populations even when they are described in pejorative terms as dying or dead. To argue to the contrary is not simply tantamount to promoting retail gentrification: it's to perpetuate negative stereotypes of the British working class, their tastes and their cultures. Indeed, it's apparent that the discourses circling around some of the most vilified and contested spaces on our High Street—e.g. fast food takeaways, late-night off-licences, tattoo parlours, betting shops, lap dance clubs—are thinly veiled expressions of class resentment, disgust and abjection. Such outlets can provide local jobs and revenue and sustain High Streets, yet this is often forgotten in rhetoric figuring them as *obstacles* to regeneration. Tellingly, these outlets are often portrayed as the haunt not of the 'respectable' working class of yesteryear, but a much derided and demonized 'chav' underclass—a 'benefit-dependent' population whose lack of taste is indicated in its appetite for fast food, cheap alcohol, popular entertainment and fake designer labels. Such characterizations are not just inaccurate, but symbolically violent. As Owen Jones (2012) argues in his brilliantly polemic *Chavs: the demonization of the working class*, by portraying the working class as inherently ignorant, successive governments have deflected attention from the real causes of social and economic inequality (and poverty) in Britain. The idea that the High Streets occupied by the less affluent need to be 'improved' is then part of the same neoliberal discourse which argues that the 'feckless' and 'addicted' classes need to be civilized because 'welfare-dependent' and 'broken' families are causing society to crumble (Jensen 2013; Wilkinson 2013; Slater 2014).

In this book, I develop this argument by considering the ways that contemporary working-class identities are being mapped onto, and out of, devalued spaces on the High Street through processes of moralization that are performative of class identities. In noting this disingenuous coupling of High Street 'decline' and the behaviour of a discredited working class, I alight on the importance of disgust as both an embodied middle-class response to, and representational trope depicting, working-class life. Disgust may seem a strong adjective to describe the emotional reaction some express towards the contemporary High Street, but it precisely communicates the dominant middle-class discourse surrounding a High Street portrayed as neither safe, clean or civilized enough to appeal to the 'mass affluent'. It's this notion of wanting to cleanse the High Street of the traces of the discredited working class that, consciously or otherwise, seems to inform much of the rhetoric of those arguing for regeneration, albeit this is frequently obscured in a language referring to 'community-led' regeneration.

Throughout this book, I combine a critical reading of national policy documents with original empirical observations and data derived from a number of research projects conducted over the last two decades in varied towns and cities. In these, I have focused on the premises often most vilified by those arguing for regeneration: the lap dance clubs, bargain booze outlets, betting shops, hot food takeaways and discount stores said to 'blight' British High Streets. While dominant discourses suggest a high level of antipathy towards such venues, my research has sought to expose the extent to which opposition is based on moral judgments of value bearing little relation to the actual social and economic role such premises play on local shopping streets. Here, I have drawn much sustenance from retail geography, which has in recent times moved beyond a fixation with the collision of culture and capital in 'spectacular spaces' to study less celebrated and even marginalized spaces such as the car boot fair (Gregson et al. 2002), charity shops (Fitton 2013), street markets (Watson and Studdert 2006), and spaces of ad hoc retail (Hunt 2015). At the same time, I've also been much inspired by work on the experience of 'ordinary' towns and small cities (e.g. Bell and Jayne 2009), turning away from London to explore the provincial towns and cities often ignored in urban scholarship. At times, this book is then focused deliberately on the local, the banal, even the parochial. It's also grounded in a very British set of debates, and specific anxieties about class and identity in an age of austerity. But for all this, this is ultimately a book that speaks to urgent international debates concerning gentrification, community and struggles for a place. The battle for the High Street is then a battle that should resonate internationally, and across disciplines, as it's at the frontline of the gentrification wars.

References

Bell, D., & Jayne, M. (2009). Small cities? Towards a research agenda. *International Journal of Urban and Regional Research, 33*(3), 683–699.

Bridge, G., & Dowling, R. (2001). Microgeographies of retailing and gentrification. *Australian Geographer, 32*(1), 93–107.

Butler, T., & Lees, L. (2006). Super-gentrification in Barnsbury, London: Globalization and gentrifying global elites at the neighbourhood level. *Transactions of the Institute of British Geographers, 31*(4), 467–487.

Coles, B. F., & Crang, P. (2011). Placing alternative consumption: Commodity fetishism in Borough Fine Foods Market, London. In T. Lewis & E. Potter (Eds.), *Ethical consumption: A critical introduction*. London: Routledge.

Davidson, M., & Wyly, E. (2012). Class-ifying London: Questioning social division and space claims in the post-industrial metropolis. *City, 16*(4), 395–421.

Deener, A. (2007). Commerce as the structure and symbol of neighborhood life: Reshaping the meaning of community in Venice, California. *City & Community, 6*(4), 291–314.

Dines, N. (2009). The disputed place of ethnic diversity: An ethnography of the redevelopment of a street market in East London. In R. Imrie, L. Lees, & M. Raco (Eds.), *Regenerating London: Governance, sustainability and community in a global city*. London: Routledge.

Fitton, T. (2013). The quite economy at a UK Charity Shop. University at York, Unpublished PhD thesis.

Freeman, L. (2011). *There goes the hood: views at gentrification from the ground up*. Philadelphia: Temple University Press.

Goetz, E. G. (2003). *Clearing the way: Deconcentrating the poor in urban America*. Chicago: The Urban Institute.

Gonzalez, S., & Waley, P. (2012). Traditional retail markets: The new gentrification frontier? *Antipode, 45*(4), 965–983.

Gotham, K. F. (2005). Tourism gentrification: The case of New Orleans' vieux carre (French Quarter). *Urban Studies, 42*(7), 1099–1121.

Gregson, N., Crewe, L., & Brooks, K. (2002). Shopping, space, and practice. *Environment and Planning (D)—Society and Space, 20*(5), 597–618.

Halnon, K. B. (2002). Poor chic: The rational consumption of poverty. *Current Sociology, 50*(4), 501–516.

Hunt, M. (2015). Keeping shop, shaping place: The vernacular curation of London's *ad hoc* consumption spaces. PhD, Royal Holloway, University of London.

Jager, M. (1986). Class definition and the aesthetics of gentrification: Victoriana in Melbourne. In N. Smith & P. Williams (Eds.), *Gentrification of the City*. Allen & Unwin: Boston, MA.

Jensen, T. (2013). Austerity parenting. *Soundings: A Journal of Politics and Culture, 55*(1), 60–70.

Jones, O. (2012). *Chavs: The demonization of the working class*. London: Verso.

Kasinitz, P., & Zukin, S. (2016). From ghetto to global: Two neighbourhood shopping streets in New York City. In S. Zukin, P. Kasinitz, & X. Chen (Eds.), *Global cities, local streets*. New York: Routledge.

Kavetsos, G. (2012). The impact of the London Olympics announcement on property prices. *Urban Studies, 49*(7), 1453–1470.

Kearns, A., & Mason, P. (2013). Defining and measuring displacement: Is relocation from restructured neighbourhoods always unwelcome and disruptive? *Housing Studies, 28*(2), 177–204.

Kern, L. (2015a). From toxic wreck to crunchy chic: Environmental gentrification through the body. *Environment and Planning D: Society and Space, 33*, 67–83.

Kleit, R. G., & Manzo, L. C. (2006). To move or not to move: Relationships to place and relocation choices in HOPE VI. *Housing Policy Debate, 17*(2), 271–308.

Lauria, M., & Knopp, L. (1985). Toward an analysis of the role of gay communities in the urban renaissance. *Urban Geography, 6*(2), 152–169.

Lees, L. (2012). The geography of gentrification: Thinking through cinoarative urbanism. *Progress in Human Geography, 36*(2), 155–171.

Lees, L., Slater, T., & Wyly, E. (2011). *Gentrification*. London: Routledge.

Ley, D. (2003). Artists, aestheticisation and the field of gentrification. *Urban Studies, 40*(12), 2527–2544.

Marcuse, P. (1985). Gentrification, abandonment and displacement: Connections, causes and policy responses in New York City. *Journal of Urban and Contemporary Law, 28*(1), 195–240.

McLean, H., Rankin, K., & Kamizaki, K. (2015). Inner-suburban neighbourhoods, activist research, and the social space of the commercial street. *ACME: An International E-Journal for Critical Geographies, 14*(4), 1283–1308.

Merrifield, A. (2013). *The new urban question*. London: Pluto Press.

Mills, C. A. (1988). "Life on the upslope": The postmodern landscape of gentrification. *Environment and Planning D: Society and Space, 6*(2), 169–189.

Moore, K. S. (2009). Gentrification in black face? The return of the black middle class to urban neighborhoods. *Urban Geography, 30*(2), 118–142.

Newman, K., & Wyly, E. K. (2006). The right to stay put, revisited: Gentrification and resistance to displacement in New York City. *Urban Studies, 43*(1), 23–57.

Paton, K. (2010). Creating the neoliberal city and citizen: The use of gentrification as urban policy in Glasgow. In N. Davidson, P. McCafferty, & D. Miller (Eds.), *Neo-liberal Scotland: Class and society in a stateless nation*. Cambridge: Cambridge Scholars Publishing.

Rankin, K. N., & McLean, H. (2015). Governing the commercial streets of the city: New terrains of disinvestment and gentrification in Toronto's inner suburbs. *Antipode, 47*(1), 216–233.

Shaw, K. (2008). Gentrification: What it is, why it is, and what can be done about it. *Geography Compass, 2*(5), 1697–1728.

Slater, T. (2014). The myth of "Broken Britain": Welfare reform and the production of ignorance. *Antipode, 46*(4), 948–969.

Smith, D. P., & Holt, L. (2007). Studentification and apprentice gentrifiers within Britain's provincial towns and cities: Extending the meaning of gentrification. *Environment and Planning A, 39*(1), 142.

Smith, N. (1996). *New urban frontier: Gentrification and the Revanchist City.* London: Routledge.

Smith, N. (2002). New globalism, new urbanism: Gentrification as global urban strategy. *Antipode, 34*(3), 427–450.

Sullivan, D. M. (2014). From food desert to food mirage: Race, social class, and food shopping in a gentrifying neighborhood. *Advances in Applied Sociology, 4*(1), 30.

Watson, S., & Studdert, D. (2006). *Markets as sites for social interaction: Spaces of diversity.* Bristol: Policy Press.

Wilkinson, E. (2013). Learning to love again: 'Broken families', citizenship and the state promotion of coupledom. *Geoforum, 49*, 206–213.

Wyly, E. (2015). Gentrification on the planetary urban frontier: The evolution of Turner's noösphere. *Urban Studies, 52*(14), 2515–2540.

Zukin, S., Kasinitz, P., & Chen, X. (2016). Spaces of everyday diversity. In S. Zukin, P. Kasinitz, & X. Chen (Eds.), *Global cities, local streets*. New York: Routledge.

Zukin, S., Trujillo, V., Frase, P., Jackson, D., Recuber, T., & Walker, A. (2009). New retail capital and neighborhood change: Boutiques and gentrification in New York City. *City & Community, 8*(1), 47–64.

2

The 'Death' of the High Street

There is a well-worn cliché suggesting Britain is a nation of shopkeepers. If this is the case, then the vitality and viability of the High Street surely provide a litmus test of the health of the nation. Standing at the metaphorical heart, but also the accessible centre, of our towns and cities, the High Street has long been idealized as the focus of community life, a lively shopping street that makes urban life at worst, bearable and, at best, immensely pleasurable. The key function of a High Street is of course, as a marketplace where goods and services are bought and sold, a site where consumers can browse before deciding to purchase. But the High Street is about more than merely shopping: it is a community space where we routinely go to meet friends, have a drink, post our letters, have our hair cut, visit a library, collect our prescriptions, perhaps take in a movie or some theatre; space in which to stroll, saunter or just hang out.

Or, at least it was. Dominant discourses now depict the High Street in Britain as in crisis. In the wake of the 2009 recession, a shallow recovery in 2010, and the threat of a 'double dip' in early 2011, many High Streets were left characterized by large numbers of boarded-up and vacant retail premises, creating a challenging operating environment for those who remained. In 2012—a veritable *annus horribilis* for the UK

© The Editor(s) (if applicable) and The Author(s) 2017
P. Hubbard, *The Battle for the High Street*,
DOI 10.1057/978-1-137-52153-8_2

retail trade—more than 750 branches of *Clintons Cards*, 611 of *Peacocks* fashion stores, 600 *Game* computer games outlets, 550 *Blockbuster* DVD rental stores, 300 *Blacks* outdoor and camping stores, 239 *HMV* stores, 187 branches of *Jessops* photography stores, and 180 *JJB Sports* stores closed, hot on the heels of the disappearance in 2009 of one of the most established of all British High Street retailers, *Woolworths* (over 800 UK stores). Combined, these closures left a legacy of vacant units (Fig. 2.1), but declining rentals and empty shop units also provided new opportunities for retailers whose business appears to be built on targeting the marginal and disadvantaged. Tellingly, the fastest growing sectors on the High Street are now 'value' retailers such as charity shops, discounters and second-hand stores (a 12% year on year increase between 2012 and 2013) and pawnbrokers, payday lenders and cheque-cashing centres (a 17% remarkable increase in the same period): other notable increases include the growth of 'ethnic' grocery and convenience stores,

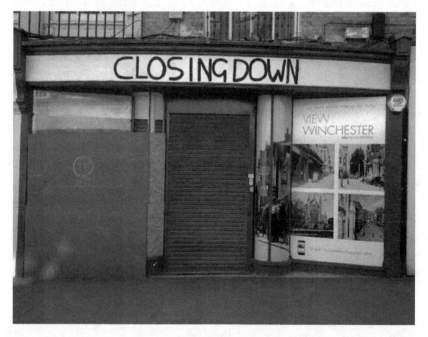

Fig. 2.1 A familiar sight on the British High Street (photo: author)

nail and tanning salons and betting shops (see Grimsey 2013). For many commentators, these discount and ad hoc stores are taking advantage of cheap rents and are of doubtful longevity. They are imagined to be very different from the 'family' businesses—e.g. grocers, butchers, bakers, and hardware stores—that once provided the mainstays of local shopping streets, and none appear to 'anchor' the High Street in quite the same way *Woolworths* once did.

Anxieties about the decline of the British High Street have generated extensive media coverage over the last decade. While some reports note larger retail centres like Leeds, Manchester and Glasgow are adapting to changing circumstances, most prognoses of the health of the High Street are much less optimistic, suggesting the rise of out-of-town lifestyles, Internet shopping and the recession have delivered a series of fatal blows. In 2000, the proportion of retail spending captured by the High Street was around 50%: by 2014, it was less than 40%, with online shopping growing in popularity. In the same year, it was estimated there were as many as 40,000 vacant properties on the High Street, or 14% of available retail units (Hughes and Jackson 2015). The fear is that these on-going processes of decline, left alone, will precipitate a mass abandonment that will leave many local shopping streets threadbare and irrelevant in the context of increasingly privatized and segmented cities where much economic and social life is online, not grounded in the physical spaces in which urban life has long been conducted.

These transformations have appeared rapid in the context of High Streets often been understood as characterized by slow change and gradual adaptation, with the media fixating on some of the most dramatic examples of decline. Among these, Margate is one of the most frequently cited. In February 2010, the Local Data Company suggested it was Britain's most empty High Street, with 27% of shops vacant. Though once the most important shopping centre in the Thanet region of East Kent, the town has seemingly suffered more than neighbouring Ramsgate and Broadstairs in terms of retail decline, with the 2005 opening of the 475,000 square foot regional shopping centre Westwood Cross (some three miles distant from Margate) precipitating a decline in footfall and a rapid rise in retail vacancies:

> There are few places more poignant than Britain's dying seaside towns, and Margate may be the saddest of all…Letters have fallen off business names—the R in *Primark*, and the N in bingo—as if the effort of clinging on to the crumbling façades was too much. On the High Street, charity shops seem to be thriving, but not much else … So forlorn is the town's retail centre that a group of A-level students walk around with clipboards, marking off the closed shops as part of their geography coursework. (Saner 2011: np)

In this sense, High Streets like Margate's that one generation ago were characterized by a 'healthy' mix of chain multiples and independents now appear to be blighted by a combination of empty shops, discount outlets and businesses depicted as only making a marginal contribution to social and economic life.

We can contrast this with the rise of new, spectacular spaces such as Westfield Stratford City, a shopping centre of nearly 2,000,000 square feet promoted as representing all that is vibrant and vital about young, multicultural Britain, situated just a short distance from the Olympic Park that provided the focus for London 2012. In the words of the developers, 'Stratford is a new metropolitan capital for East London, a city within a city, an innovative and dynamic place for a new generation of consumers to shop, to eat, to meet, to be entertained and to stay' (Westfield City 2011). While this is boosterist marketing rhetoric of the most obvious kind, even hardened academics can be beguiled by the sensory pleasures and disorientations associated with this new 'public' space. Myria Georgiou (2013), for example, approvingly notes that the centre boasts well-known high-status fashion brands, familiar through global mediation, but also houses lower-price stores and familiar fast food franchises, a diversification of experience assumed to mirror the tastes and pockets of visitors to this modern agora. Whatever, the rise of spectacular retail developments such as Westfield Stratford City only exacerbates the sense of decline on High Streets like Margate's, suggesting there is little basis for optimism about the future of some local shopping streets.

Margate and Westfield of course represent extremes: one, a contrived and carefully planned retail spectacle benefitting from its proximity to London's Olympic Park, the other, a 'gap toothed' High Street in a seaside town largely forgotten and unloved by a British public that has moved on from its love affair with the 'kiss me quick' bucket-and-spade holiday. However, I will return to both subsequently, not because they are necessarily representative, but precisely because they are taken as indicative of shifts in society and space casting doubt over the sustainability of the 'traditional' High Street. But these are not the only symbolic places which recur in the narrative of High Street decline, as almost all small cities and towns can boast their own stories of stagnation and decline, or speak of the malign influence of a newly minted regional shopping centre. The narratives are of course geographically contingent and take pronounced forms in the more struggling regions. For example, in the less prosperous North and Midlands, secondary retail centres have been particularly badly hit by the recession, with around one in six retail premises standing vacant on the average High Street. As such, it was not especially surprising when, in 2012, Margate's crown as Britain's most vacant High Street was snatched by Hartlepool, which in turn lost its unenviable title to Burslem (Stoke on Trent) in 2015. By then, more than 10,000 shops in the UK had remained empty for more than three years (Local Data Company 2015).

Regenerating the High Street

In the wake of the recession, the regeneration of the High Street has become a matter of considerable public and policy debate, with a slew of initiatives and reports emerging which offer potential solutions to its perceived decline. These are by no means consensual. Differences of opinion are evident, for example, about whether some shrinkage of the High Street is desirable, a pressing issue in the context of the acute shortage of affordable housing in much of the UK: converting disused shops into new housing seems both expedient and sensible in cases when the High Street shows little sign of revival. Indeed, some see the replacement of shops by housing, as well as education, arts, health and office space, as the obvious answer to what is often described as a structural over-supply of retail space (see Carmona 2014). However, such shrinkage is not accepted as inevitable by all, with many still holding to the ideals of the High Street as the focus of retail activity, albeit perhaps better integrated with the changing landscapes of online and e-retailing (Digital High Street Advisory Board 2015). Yet, even among those who see opportunities to attract back vibrant retail businesses to the High Street, it is acknowledged that there is not one simple answer to retail regeneration, as the solutions which work are felt to be 'as divergent as the retail marketplace', needing to be 'tailored to local opportunities' (Grimsey 2013: 5).

Despite points of disagreement, there is a consensus that vacant shops are undesirable, with long-term retail vacancies creating a physical and social stigma that can result in a cycle of decline. In her influential Review of British High Streets, commissioned by the coalition government, self-styled 'retail guru' Mary Portas (2011) teases out these relationships, presenting a causal process in which the falling demand for some goods is strongly shaped by the economic and social character of a local area, which in turn influences retailers' perceptions of the vitality of a retail location. The retrenchment of certain retail chains and their focus on more viable and 'functional' locations creates 'economic obsolescence' in some local retail areas, with shrinkage in retail floorspace being the most obvious symptom. This creates a downwards spiral with dereliction in both cause and effect:

> When important properties in the middle of High Streets are empty it pulls down the attractiveness and desirability of the street. The problems associated with empty properties are considerable. They attract vandalism and increase insecurity and fear. And this all reduces the value of surrounding businesses and homes. So the decision to leave a property empty is not just a private matter for the landlord. It affects us all. Innovative solutions could add value to not just the individual properties but to the surrounding area. (Portas 2011: 35)

Others agree that unsightly, empty and abandoned shops repel potential shoppers. For example, deploying a (widely discredited) logic inherited from the 'broken windows' thesis of environmental criminology, Paul Swinney and Dmitry Sivaev (2013) suggest empty shops are not just eyesores, but have the potential to attract crime and anti-social behavior. Similarly, the London Assembly's (2013) report on the capital's High Streets suggests these can precipitate a 'vicious circle' in which a rise in empty shops discourages people from visiting an area, reducing the potential customer base and causing further vacancies.

Encouraging the re-use of vacant premises is then an important theme in policy discourse, with the rise of charity shops one symptom given Business Rates are waived for charities (Paget and Birdwell 2013, reporting a 30% increase in charity shops on the British High Street in the preceding five years). Yet, in some accounts charity shops are regarded as only a temporary solution to the empty shop problem, dismissed as a transient sticking plaster that does little to restore the vitality and viability of the High Street. Some have even suggested that these stores do more harm than good by driving down rentals, and lump these together with other 'unwanted' High Street outlets:

> Town centres … are becoming swamped with payday lenders, pawnbrokers and pound shops. As our High Streets become increasingly geared towards making money from people who don't have any, shoppers with disposable income are going elsewhere—and so are big name retailers. Things aren't looking good for my hometown of Rochdale. Even *McDonald's* fled the High Street in 2011 after "seeing trading patterns in the town centre change". Since then, many other big names have followed suit. The shop unit where *McDonald's* once stood is still vacant. Next door a nameless discount store has sprung up, and *B&M Bargains* has opened up across the street. Nearby, a charity shop sits alongside a pawnbrokers. There is a *Quicksilver* arcade next door, followed by *Pound Zone*, with two more charity shops opposite. Further up, *The Money Shop* stands opposite *Cash Generator*, and most of the surrounding units are closed or vacant. (Speak 2013: np)

For Rochdale, also read Margate, Hartlepool or Burslem, Or Rotherham, Walsall and Preston, Or Whitechapel High Street, Chrisp Street in Tower Hamlets and the other local shopping streets in London typified by high levels of vacancy and 'betting shops, pawnbrokers and down-market fast food takeaways which frighten shoppers away' (Greater London Authority 2013: 5).

Time and again, clusters of discount stores, fast food restaurants, money lenders and betting shops have been cited by policymakers, town centre managers and local authorities as 'lowering the tone' of the High Street, with their replacement by a diverse mix of independent, up-market stores idealized as a positive route to retail revival (Coca-Stefaniak 2013). When coupled with a solid retail partnership between the private and public sector, it is these independent stores imagined as the virtuous businesses whose clientele will bring renewed waves of investment to the High Street and return it to its former glories (British Retail Consortium 2009). It is here that the logic of Town Centre Management schemes and Business Improvement Districts (BIDS) becomes clearer; rather than merely halting the downwards spiral of vacancy and blight, these aim to regenerate the High Street by attracting new visitors, widening the client base of the High Street through an overt targeting of the middle classes. Aesthetic improvements—no matter how superficial—are used to reverse images of decline. New businesses, preferably independent and locally owned, are courted, sometimes offered vacant premises, at heavily discounted rentals. Art galleries, vintage boutiques and cafés are privileged, alongside other 'healthy' facilities that can bestow users with some form of educational, cultural or social capital. 'Pop-up' shops abound. Traditional street markets are updated, re-launched as 'Farmers' Markets'. 'Family-oriented' activities, fun days and seasonal events are used as bait to lure new consumers, as is late night shopping and free or cheap parking.

Media discourses about the state of the High Street repeatedly present such solutions as commonsensical. We are told the High Street is dying and can only be revived through the attraction of independent, 'community-oriented' stores which will replace the payday lenders, charity shops, fast food restaurants, bookmakers, cut-price stores and sex shops which are 'swamping' High Streets. In the words of Bill Grimsey, a former butcher's boy and retail entrepreneur, many High Streets have become overwhelmed by such outlets, something that means they are 'as good as dead already'. Advocating changes to business rates to revive High Street fortunes, he argued:

> We want to avoid just having more charity shops, more payday loan shops, more betting shops, all of which are preying on the poor in our society—because what is a payday loan shop? A place to get access to funds. What is a betting shop? It is a place to live your dream in hope. What is a charity shop? It is a place to get cheap items. Are we really satisfied that is the

legacy that we are producing for our grandchildren, up and down the country? (Grimsey, oral evidence to Business, Innovation and Skills committee, 29 August 2013: 37)

Following the election of 2010, various Coalition politicians agreed with Grimsey that reviving the High Street required joined-up governance, including (according to then-Business Secretary Vince Cable) revised business rates for small shops, and, in the view of Planning Minister Nick Boles, the revision of existing planning and licensing laws to enable more control over the type of businesses allowed on the High Street. When introducing controls designed to ensure all new betting shops have to apply for planning permission, the latter argued that the 'government is taking action to support healthy and vibrant local High Streets' putting 'empty and redundant buildings back into productive use and making it easier for valued town centre businesses like shops, banks and cafés to open new premises, while giving councils greater powers to tackle the harm to local amenity caused by a concentration of particular uses' (cited in Bird 2014: 1). Alongside changes to permitted development rights and tax breaks for shops, the Coalition government also set up a High Street Innovation Fund (worth £10 million) to help local authorities with empty premises and especially those High Streets most affected by the 2011 English 'riots'. Additionally, it launched the Great British High Street Awards in 2014 to acknowledge the progress made by some towns in reversing the decline.

These policy initiatives underlined the Coalition's government's commitment to a High Street that could be described 'as the veins and arteries' that keep the hearts of towns and cities beating (DCLG 2012: 3). Significantly, all espoused variants of 'community-led' regeneration, with Housing and Planning Minister Brandon Lewis (2013: 2) stressing 'it's local communities who know what makes their High Street unique and can capitalise on those retail strengths to build a sense of loyalty and pride among locals'. It was this logic that underpinned the government's commissioning of the Portas Review in 2011. Making 28 broad recommendations, including many supporting independent retailers, Mary Portas' report has subsequently provided the touchstone for town centre renewal in England and Wales in which local communities are identified as key agents in the making of vibrant, attractive and inclusive High Streets: the first tranche of 'Portas Pilot' towns included 12 'failing' High Streets—Bedford, Bedminster, Croydon, Dartford, Liskeard, Margate, Market Rasen, Nelson, Newbiggin, Stockport, Stockton and Wolverhampton—each underpinned by a 'town team' charged with coming up with a visionary, strategic and operational plan. The aim of these pilot projects was not simply to generate income for retailers, but to create 'lively, dynamic, exciting and social places that give a sense of belonging and trust to a community' (Portas 2011: 2). A key activity here has been the re-use of vacant retail units, with local organizations developing 'pop-up' shops designed to dispel perceptions of decline and to attract new shoppers and visitors (Ferreri 2016). Here, there is an obvious enthusiasm for initiatives promoting the new vernacular of creativity—craft stores, vintage shops, community cafés, temporary art galleries—all dressed up in the stripped-back shabby chic aesthetic of austerity nostalgia.

The promotion of 'community-led' High Street regeneration has been a matter of agreement across political divides, with the shadow government arguing in its policy review of retail regeneration that

> Healthy High Streets offer something that shopping centres and Internet sites, though quick and convenient, cannot; a sense of character and individuality that reflects the people that live there and makes them proud of their area. We want to give communities the tools they need to create these kinds of sustainable places that will keep people coming back week after week and attract investment and jobs to the centre of our towns and cities. That is why Labour wants to give communities greater powers to stop the clustering of certain types of premises, such as payday loan companies, and support locally-led diversification of High Streets and town centres. (Labour Policy Review 2012: 5)

Again, here the rhetoric emphasizes the importance of not just ensuring empty shops are bought back into use, but replacing the existing businesses thought to 'blight' High Streets with a more diverse range of 'community-oriented' facilities. This type of assertion was mirrored in Scotland by the commissioning of a National Review of Town Centres ('The Fraser Review'), an arguably more expansive document than the Portas Review, which stated that 'in many town centres there is an abundance of empty and abandoned property that community organizations could beneficially occupy' (External Advisory Group 2013: 11).

Scottish Planning Policy was altered in 2014 to reflect this, setting out a 'town centres first' policy designed to attract significant numbers of people back to town centres by encouraging a healthy mix of retail, commercial and cultural facilities back into struggling town centres.

Challenging this bi-partisan and cross-border political consensus is difficult. However, that is precisely what this book sets out to do. At the heart of my argument is the contention that the dominant discourse around High Street regeneration is essentially class-laden, and should—indeed, must—be contested. Writing from the perspective of a critical social scientist, I find the notion that High Streets must cater to the 'community at large' or be 'community-oriented' problematic in the extreme. As generations of sociologists and geographers have noted, 'community' is a term carrying connotations of social belonging, collective well-being, solidarity and support, but this always being conditional on exclusion of those perceived not to belong. In the words of Iris Marion Young (1990: 314), the usual idea of community seeks to suppress difference, contrary to the ideals of 'city life as an openness to unassimilated otherness'. This hints at the fractured nature of contemporary urban society: despite governmental efforts to engineer cohesive communities based on multiculturalism and inclusion, communities in practice are typically defined in relation to 'otherness' (i.e. defined in relation to those who are excluded from belonging to it). In this light, it is hard to talk of the 'community at large': within each city there is not one community but potentially several. Indeed, empirical study suggests the contemporary British city is often starkly divided between different class factions or taste communities, with these groups often living separate lives, a result of processes of residential segregation in which the affluent inhabit increasingly divergent social universes from those below them in the social hierarchy (see Dorling and Rees 2003; Davidson and Wyly 2012; Fenton et al. 2013). In spite of this, High Street regeneration agendas are based upon a utopian vision of universalized upward mobility that identifies no necessary socio-economic antagonisms, ignoring the realities of a divided society where different populations consume differently. Dominant ideas of retail regeneration are then predicated on the fiction of a High Street 'for all' in which certain up-market businesses are approved, but others—typically those frequented by the less affluent—are deemed unhealthy, unwanted or even toxic.

Keep Calm and Eat Cupcakes: Retail Policy in Austerity Britain

The emergence of discount stores and payday lenders on the British High Street is one of the most palpable symptoms of a recession that has left the poorest in society less able to afford the goods and services, which the wealthier regard as normal. If one considers the 'decline' of many High Streets in this light, their changing form can be seen as a result of recessionary pressures, benefit reductions and a widening gulf between the affluent and the marginal. But at times retail policy seems to forget this, ignoring the diverse ways that local shopping streets are produced and consumed by the working poor, the unemployed, recent migrants, asylum seekers and so on. Rather than focusing on their needs and the way declining High Streets need to adapt to recessionary times, many policy missives instead focus on the middle classes, and how the High Street meets their tastes and aspirations. While this focus is not especially surprising given the way that the British media refracts and reflects middle-class opinion, it is a dangerously narrow perspective to be taken, given that the strains experienced among sections of the (struggling) middle class appear to be leading to feelings of moral indignation or 'ressentiment' routinely expressed in the form of a moralizing social reaction (Le Grand, 2015). As Owen Jones (2012) shows, in recessionary Britain, this has taken a variety of malicious forms, most notably the demonization of white working-class populations—'chavs'—whose individual moral failings are deemed responsible for the fragmentation not only of their own communities but Britain as a whole. But this spurious reasoning and scapegoating goes further than this, with the decline of the British High Street also linked to poisonous rhetoric that blames the corrosion of British character on the arrival of particular migrant communities. While such migrants or 'ethnic entrepreneurs' are often heralded as respectable, hard-working and community-minded populations, we will see in this book that businesses perceived to be catering for 'ethnic communities' are seldom described as part of the 'good' High Street, and often depicted as a malign presence.

In this light, many of the prescriptions for the revival of the High Street appear inherently nostalgic, harkening back to an imagined era when the High Street served all in society, and local shopping streets propped up the myth of a more equal post-war society (Watson and Wells 2005). This is certainly to the fore in Mary Portas' autobiography of growing up in the 1960s Rickmansworth, *Shop Girl*, where she speaks of shops as:

> Places where the bell always pings as you open the door, the air hits you warm as you walk inside and a smile greets you. Most of all, they are places where people chat and collect news, exchange gossip and advice, meet, greet and love—or sometimes hate—their neighbours. Even as a six-year-old, I know there is a world enclosed in the four tiny letters of the word 'shop'. (Portas 2015: 3)

Elsewhere she speaks of the importance of local shopkeepers in supporting her family when her mother died when she was aged 16, suggesting the 'faceless mutes' found behind the contemporary supermarket till could not fulfill the same function (Portas 2010: np). As she puts it, 'in a world where some of the most efficient shopping is now online and supermarkets have killed off the final vestiges of human contact through the questionable benefits of "self scanning", it's the remaining shops on our High Streets that for many of us represent some of our most important social interaction' (Portas 2010: np). This condemnation of the lack of meaningful human contact evident in the contemporary retail landscape is not uncommon, with frequent reference made in policy discussions to the value of the personal attention that was paid to the customer in years gone by. Oddly, this type of discourse is also entwined with memories of a simpler, thriftier time, where the Sunday roast stretched to Monday's bubble and squeak, and Shepherd's Pie on a Tuesday, 'if there was still enough left' (Portas 2015: 23). This is a language in keeping with the mood of the recessionary times, given wartime rationing, the values of thrift and the virtues of recycling ('make do and mend') have become the subject of nostalgic longing, and hence highly valued in food, fashion and design (Jackson 2016).

On this basis, it is tempting to suggest that policy for the High Street is not so much concerned with addressing the decline of High Streets as preserving a particular notion of the 'Great British' High Street. Indeed, strategies intended to increase the vitality and viability of the High Street seem to be preoccupied with blaming the poor and minorities for the dissatisfactions of the present, spelling out strategies designed to make High

Street more attractive for those middle-class consumers who have generally shunned local shopping streets in favour of online and out-of-town retailing, but could be tempted back by the promise of a more 'authentic', bespoke experience rooted in images of the High Street of yesteryear. The key here has been the promotion of the independently owned 'local' businesses, with the type of 'austerity nostalgia' (Hatherley 2016) espoused by Portas encouraging shabby chic vintage shops, hipster micropubs and retro cupcake shops over the mix of chain-owned pound and 99p stores, 'ethnic stores', betting shops, charity shops and tanning centres taken to epitomize failing High Streets.

In many policy documents, the presence of independently owned stores is hence taken as the key barometer of the vitality of a High Street, and a sign of local revival. This conflation of the independent with the local or authentic is, as we shall see, highly problematic. Irrespective, in reports compiled by the New Economics Foundation, the move from being a 'clone town' (dominated by multiples) to a 'hometown' (dominated by independently owned businesses) is described as cause for celebration:

> A hometown is a place that retains its individual character and is instantly recognizable and distinctive to the people who live there, as well as those who visit. A clone town is a place that has had the individuality of its High Street shops replaced by a monochrome strip of global and national chains that means its retail heart could easily be mistaken for dozens of other bland town centres across the country. (New Economics Foundation 2003: 4)

The New Economics Foundation (2010) heralded Whitstable in Kent as the highest scoring town in terms of its proportion of independent stores, with this described as the outcome of efforts to improve its local distinctiveness and create a sustainable local food culture. What is not noted is that over the period 2005–2010, Whitstable was one of the most rapidly gentrifying towns on the south coast, with the rise of local businesses tied into incomers' obvious appetite for seafood, vintage fashions, and 'proper' coffee (Kennell 2011). Indeed, the independent stores that have blossomed in Whitstable are not the independent grocers or convenience stores that characterized the town's High Street in the 1970s and 1980s, but a range of bijou and self-consciously twee outlets: *Buttercup Boutique*, with its award-winning wooden toys, kitsch gift shop *Taking the Plunge*, the *Cheese Box*, boasting artisanal cheese, and so on (Fig. 2.2). These regularly receive celebrity endorsements, with Janet Street Porter (2012) raving in *The Daily Telegraph* about 'quirky little independently run shops' and suggesting a trip to the *Whitstable Oyster Stores* (baked halibut £23, cod and chips £16.50) is not to be missed. The celebratory tone of the New Economics Foundation's conclusion that the rise of independently owned stores is evidence of 'communities fighting back' needs to be tempered with acknowledgment that articulate, middle-class communities are those most able to create a High Street meeting their aspirations: while locally owned shops are perfectly capable of supporting a range of tastes and pockets, in many instances they are oriented towards more affluent consumers and visitors.

There has been very little academic assessment of what the consequences of the 'boutiquing' of the High Street are for different social groups. This is surprising, given that the 'disadvantaged consumer' was a major figure in the retail geography of the 1980s and 1990s (see Guy 1985; Sparks

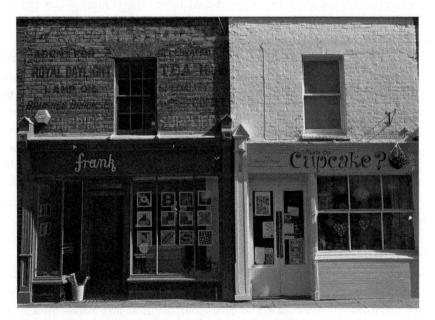

Fig. 2.2 Boutiquing, Whitstable, Kent (photo: author)

1987; Westlake and Dagleish 1990; Bromley and Thomas 1995; Williams and Hubbard 2001). Indeed, in the wake of what was termed the 'third wave' of retail decentralization (involving the co-location of warehouse retailers and supermarkets on out-of-town retail parks surrounding most major towns) (Schiller 1986), much of the work in the sub-discipline was preoccupied with identifying which groups exhibited spatially constrained patterns of shopping behaviour, frequenting local shopping streets rather than venturing to newer out-of-town facilities. The overwhelming conclusion of such work was that there was an increasing divide between the mobile (who were mostly younger and more affluent) and the relatively immobile (including the poor, the disabled, and the elderly), with the former being more spatially expansive in terms of their routine shopping behaviours. So while the more affluent took advantage of the newer facilities, others remained reliant on the older (and sometimes declining) range of shops on the High Street. Increasing numbers appeared unable to enjoy the benefits of the so-called *retail revolution*.

The notion of the disadvantaged consumer stressed shopping behavior could, to some extent, be predicted by an individual's social status, with consumer disadvantage strongly linked to wider dynamics of social exclusion. However, some deferred, arguing consumer disadvantage could not always be understood in terms of the traditional sociological categories of class and income. For instance, in a study of the retail habits of Coventry consumers conducted in the late 1990s, we noted that age and car ownership were better predictors of grocery-shopping behavior than household income per se (Williams and Hubbard 2001). Likewise, Rosemary Bromley and Colin Thomas (1995) found only 38% of carless households in Swansea frequented superstores, in contrast to 67% of car-owning households. This focus on access and the importance of car ownership stressed that place of residence, and relative distance from stores, could be as important as socio-economic deprivation in producing disadvantage. Irrespective, an important conclusion of research into retail disadvantage was that the inability to utilize the newer, out-of-town stores was something impacting on quality of life, with particular concerns voiced about the inability of some populations to obtain clothing, essential household goods and food and drink at affordable prices. In some neighbourhoods, the closure of greengrocers, butchers and bakers left isolated 'cornershops' or garage forecourt shops the only possible local source of groceries, with these often selling inferior goods at higher prices than their out-of-town counterparts. It led to some areas of British cities being labelled 'food-deserts' as increasing problems of nutrition become apparent (see, inter alia, Cummins and Macintyre 1999; Wrigley et al. 2002; Guy et al. 2004).

While Internet shopping (via *Amazon* and its ilk) arguably assuaged some of the earlier concerns voiced about peoples' ability to access to comparison goods, the availability of fresh fruit and vegetables hence remained an important focus of retail studies into the twenty-first century. Here, the identification of a national 'obesity panic' (see Chap. 9) gave fresh impetus to studies focused on the links between socio-economic status, diet and body mass, with one of the main predictors of obesity—reliance on fast food with high calorific content—appearing related to the lack of affordable fruit and vegetables in more deprived communities. The fact that this has been connected to the locational strategies of the 'big four' supermarket chains who dominated food retailing in the UK from the 1990s onwards—i.e. *Tesco, Sainsburys, Asda* and *Safeway/Morrisons*—was underlined in Neil Wrigley et al.'s (2002) study of the Seacroft estate in Leeds. This account of a 'food desert' before and after the opening of a *Tesco* superstore nearby revealed that 45% of residents switched to the new store as their main source for food once it opened, with the fruit and vegetable consumption of those who did so increasing by an average of 2.5 portions per week.

Over time, researchers' concern with consumer disadvantage has been replaced by a more specific focus on access to foodstuffs (Bromley and Matthews 2007). But even here, the debate became somewhat muted, with the rediscovery of the High Street by the UK's most important food retailers (particularly in the form of *Tesco Metro* and *Express* stores, as well as *Sainsbury's Local*) ostensibly mitigating some of the most pernicious effects of retail restructuring. These retailers have been astute in recognizing that growing numbers of consumers are not convinced by the merits of weekly out-of-town food shopping, and instead seek convenience at the local/community scale (Wrigley and Brookes 2015). This re-localization of food shopping into the town centre has had important implications for some High Streets, with these corporate convenience stores becoming the anchor of many smaller town centres. The empirical research on the new generation of corporate convenience stores is as yet sparse, but unquestionably the arrival of these stores has provided new shopping options for those previously unable (or unwilling) to access out-of-town stores. Wrigley et al. (2007), for example, found the opening of a *Tesco Express* in St Mary's—a disadvantaged inner city district in Southampton—resulted in a 50% increase in residents using a local store for their primary shopping trip for groceries, as opposed to the other alternative, a mile-long journey to an Asda superstore. Another Southampton-based study—Lucy Woodliffe's (2004: 17) study of the suburb of Shirley, where there is both a *Tescos Express* and small *Sainsburys* on the High Street—goes so far to question the whole notion of consumer disadvantage, differentiating between the elderly, large families, the unemployed, low-income earners, ethnic minorities, lone parents and other 'marginally disadvantaged' groups and those suffering what Woodliffe terms 'extreme disadvantage' because of severe personal mobility problems (including the physically disabled and those with limiting long-term illnesses). Describing the latter as 'neglected' consumers, she essentially refines the notion of retail disadvantage by implying only those with debilitating personal circumstances have been negatively affected by retail change since the 1980s.

The evidence suggesting the poorer in society have been profoundly disadvantaged by retail change, and specifically by the development of out-of-town shopping, is then far from unequivocal. Nevertheless, the focus on the disadvantaged consumer in retail studies was one that, for a long time, fitted in well with a story suggesting the success of out-of-town retailing had occurred to the detriment of the High Street and the consumers that relied on it. Indeed, there is little doubt that academic studies on retail disadvantage proved influential in prompting the more restrictive planning policies discouraging out-of-town retailing emerging from the 1990s onwards (Findlay and Sparks 2009). The inability of declining High Streets and 'secondary retail centres' to cater for the needs of the poor, immobile, and those experiencing forms of social disadvantage was certainly among the key factors that encouraged the emergence of a 'town centre first' policy (enshrined in the government's Planning Policy Guidance Note 6, 1993) which suggested out-of-town retail was only acceptable in situations where it would not undermine the 'vitality and viability' of nearby retail centres. The dominant idea at this time was that defending the High Street was essential given it theoretically could serve the 'whole community', unlike the out-of-town locations regarded as catering principally for more affluent, car-borne consumers. Subsequent planning policy missives all placed similar emphasis on the need to provide a wide range of retail services in environments 'accessible to all', with policy-makers remaining conscious of the evidence that poor diet is associated with peoples' inability to access, and not necessarily afford, fresh fruit and vegetables (Guy and David 2004).

However, this fixation with disadvantaged consumers and communities seemingly dissipated in the wake of the recession of 2009, which raised a more pressing series of questions about the sustainability and resilience of the High Street. A rapid collapse in consumer confidence at this time precipitated a matching lack of confidence amongst investors that many stores—and particularly comparison retailers on the High Street—had any future. For developers, the High Street suddenly lost its gloss as an attractive investment, with the numbers of shops owned by financial institutions falling as a response. With the closure of some of the most familiar stores on the British High Street, the question was no longer whether High Streets could adequately serve the less affluent, but whether they could survive at all. As we have seen, the 'death' of the High Street was mooted as a possibility, with cases such as Margate presented as prime evidence. The context here—one of 'austerity' and governmental cuts to public services—was hardly one that bred optimism, with New Labour's mantra 'things can only get better' replaced by the Coalition's refrain that things were going to get a lot worse, and that a rapid and painful retrenchment of public spending was necessary to reduce national indebtedness (Taylor-Gooby and Stoker 2011).

But has the decline of the High Street been overstated? Bearing in mind the shift towards 'convenience cultures', Wrigley and Dolega (2011) certainly think so, and point to the fact that many premises vacated in the retail recession of 2009–10, were quickly re-let. Critics have, of course, highlighted that many new stores were distinctly down-market ones targeting a less affluent clientele and privileging quantity over quality. For example, the Local Data Company reported in 2012 that one-third of the former Woolworths stores that were re-let within a year was occupied by discount stores, most notably *Poundland* but also *Home Bargains*,

Poundworld and the *99p Shop*. These typically offer a diverse range of household goods, and some groceries, alongside cut-priced confectionary, stationary and toys at 'pocket-money' prices. But far from being considered part of a vital and viable High Street, matched to the mood of austerity Britain, such stores have been lumped in with the betting shops, payday lenders, charity shops and fast food restaurants that have also been increasing in number on the post-recessionary High Streets. Few describe these in positive terms, the defence offered by Chris Gilson in *The Guardian* an all-too-rare exception:

> Take a trip down our High Street today and you would walk past a 99p shop, a *Poundland*, a *Poundworld*, a *Mr Pound*, and to the amusement of many, a 97p shop, complete with sub-quid sandwiches. And while some have laughed at a price war that starts so close to the bottom, these retailers offer something more than many of their neighbours. It seems an obvious point, but pound stores are cheap, something that is crucial in these straitened times. We fret about what will draw people to our High Streets in the wake of the loss of trade to online retailers. The popularity of cut-price shops offers an answer, though it may be an unpopular one among those yearning for the return of *Marks & Spencers* and *Woolworths* to the High Streets from which they have disappeared … Uncomfortable as that may be, the fact remains that, for many, these shops are a necessity. (Gilson 2014: np)

The implication here is that much of the concern about the health of the High Street is misplaced, and predicated on class-based anxieties about the type of stores that are actually prospering. Dismissed as variously garish, unhealthy or simply cheap, shops on 'failing' High Streets are rarely considered in terms of what they do in terms of providing services to the less affluent 'disadvantaged consumer', let alone providing jobs for local residents. Though economically viable, they are dismissed as promoting 'bad' forms of consumption, forms assumed to be off-putting for the middle classes. Somehow then, the dominant arguments have flipped round; High Streets once accused of failing to cater adequately for the disadvantaged are now condemned for having no appeal for anyone *except* the disadvantaged consumer. National retail policy is then not much concerned with the 'decline' of High Streets per se, but reinventing the High Street in ways that will ensure it appeals to the middle classes.

The fact that the prescribed measures are likely to displace the less affluent is left unacknowledged, and the threat of retail gentrification unspoken.

Retail Policy as Moralizing Discourse

Located at the interface of sociology, geography and retail studies, this book is particularly influenced by contemporary sociological literatures on class, as well as geographic ones on gentrification. In recent times, both literatures have converged around the analysis of the *language* used to condemn, and ultimately displace, working-class cultures. This book thus explores retail gentrification by focusing on the representation of High Street decline, particularly those moralizing discourses figuring certain outlets and stores as detrimental to High Street vitality and viability. These outlets are those frequently contrasted in unfavourable terms with the type of upscale retail most associated with gentrified neighbourhoods:

> In upmarket neighbourhoods many retail areas have already bounced back. Traditional retail parades of grocers, bakers and butchers have been replaced by continental bistros, coffee shops, delis and boutiques selling expensive knick-knacks. Regenerated, reinvigorated and restyled in heritage colours, they present the epitome of a modern urbane lifestyle ... In others there has been an unprecedented growth of an unhealthy, and potentially harmful, 'toxic', mix of uses. These include fast food takeaways and 'all you can eat' buffet style restaurants, selling energy-dense, nutritionally poor food; sub-prime money lenders offering instant cash and 'payday' loans at extortionate interest rates; and betting shops where traditional betting on sporting events has been almost completely supplanted by electronic gaming machines on which it's possible to gamble hundreds of pounds in minutes. To this list might be added other uses, such as tanning salons, body piercing parlours, shops selling cut price (sometimes counterfeit) alcohol and tobacco and so on. (Townshend 2016: 3)

These are the type of premises highlighted in a Local Government Association (2012) survey that reported that 52% feel the clustering of these premises has a negative effect on the High Street. Top of this list were strip clubs and sex shops, which 57% of respondents felt would have negative impacts, 50% for betting shops, 36% for fast food outlets, 36% tanning shops, 24% nail bars and 19% for pubs/bars (Local Government Association 2012). At first sight, this type of finding lends obvious support to calls for tighter planning regulation of such premises, which are accused of sapping the vitality and viability of British High Streets. Yet a closer analysis of the results shows that working-class populations (i.e. those manual and routine workers belonging to social groups 'D' and 'E') are more favourably disposed towards betting shops, tanning shops, sex shops, fast food outlets and off-licences than more affluent consumers (i.e. professionals in social groups 'A' and 'B'). And this immediately suggests that notions of value, and visions of the future High Street, are contestable as they involve the discursive devaluation of certain tastes, cultures and lifestyles, and the privileging of others. What are regarded by some as unwanted or even noxious premises are clearly valued by others, and play a role in community life despite accusations that they have little positive contribution to make. Policies predicated on inclusion thus bequeath exclusion, and—however inadvertently—end up supporting processes of retail gentrification.

Here it is worth noting that the language used by policy-makers espousing retail regeneration of our failing High Streets is inherently contradictory. On the one hand, it emphasizes the desirability of 'inclusive' High Streets, advocating safe, diverse streets with a varied mix of restaurants, libraries, banks, shops, and pubs. But on the other hand, it is deeply intolerant, with some premises routinely depicted as antithetical to the cultivation of a convivial and sustainable city. As much as promoting vibrant High Streets where there are few vacant premises, much retail policy actually seems fixated on *closing* premises. Fuelled by images of disgust, the language justifying such measures describes these businesses as not just cheap, but inherently damaging to local well-being. For example, in 2015, the Royal Society for Public Health presented research showing distinct concentrations of bookmakers, fast food takeaways, payday lenders and tanning shops in places experiencing high levels of morbidity and premature mortality (Fig. 2.3). In contrast, healthy High Streets were identified as supporting social interaction and mental well-being thanks to higher numbers of pharmacies, health centres, museums, art galleries, leisure centres and libraries. The recommendation, following that of

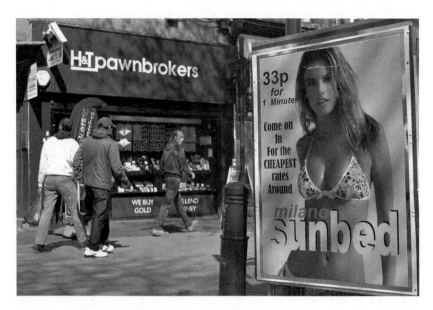

Fig. 2.3   An unhealthy High Street? (photo: author)

Mary Portas, was that tighter regulation via planning and licensing is needed to prevent High Streets being over-run by 'unhealthy' businesses.

This book takes issue with such prognoses. It does not question the assertion that some local shopping streets are used by people with generally poorer mental and physical health, but it argues that this is a function of class and deprivation. Inevitably, some High Streets are used by wealthy populations, others by the less affluent, and we know that poorer people tend to have worse health than wealthier ones (see Leventhal and Brooks-Gunn 2003). In that sense, we need to challenge the type of spurious reasoning suggesting some businesses *cause* poor health, and hence have no place on the High Street. For example, the idea that a payday lender is the cause of ill health, stress and mental illness among those who use it ignores a whole host of intervening variables, namely ones of socio-economic status and income. Who is to say that without the existence of payday lenders that the health of some might be even worse? After all, for those needing to service debts, these provide a ready source of money not offered by the High Street banks (whose closure was part of the financial abandonment that thrust many of the poor into deeper levels of indebtedness in the first place) (Leyshon and Thrift 1995). Likewise, while problematic gambling is a major social issue, bookmakers offer a space of sociality and leisure that can be important for some in maintaining a sense of identity and belonging. Similarly, while fast food is obviously associated with obesity as much of it is high in calorific content and low in nutrients, many of those who choose to eat at fast food restaurants manage to maintain healthy lifestyles (and some of these restaurants offer healthier options). And although the Royal Society of Public Health alleges the typical sunbed user is less healthy than non-users, has worse diet, drinks more and is more likely to smoke, with use of sunbeds also correlated with skin cancer in some studies (Green et al. 2007), it could be countered that the use of sunbeds in moderation is not particularly unhealthy, and can provide relaxation and positive mood effects for users who lack gardens or relaxation spaces in their own homes (Murray and Turner 2004).

The assumptions that some businesses are unhealthy or disorderly are not necessarily based on spurious correlation, as clearly there is some relationship between these outlets and the prevalence of poor and ill health in some communities. But, as the famous aphorism would have it, correlation does not equal causation. These facilities may be more present in areas where there are fewer affluent consumers present, or be more frequented by poorer residents in areas where there is a more mixed residential population, but the poor are not made poor by these facilities, or the wealth of the affluent necessarily threatened by them. The opposition to them is then, I would argue, a misguided mixture of patronizing paternalism and an outright disavowal of the British working class by the middle classes whose opinions are reflected in media and policy discourses.

So a key argument in this book is that the assumptions about healthy and valued High Streets prevalent in policy and media discourse are underpinned by middle-class assumptions about respectable behaviours and modes of interaction. Put simply, fast food takeaways, betting shops, payday lenders, tanning outlets (and so on) appear to trigger forms of repulsion among the middle class because they are seen to embody an excessive or ill-mannered working-class identity that is 'out of place' in the gentrifying city. As such, the desire to regenerate the High Street can, I argue, be best understood as an attempt to transform and re-moralize it, imbuing it with the virtues and tastes of the middle classes, displacing traces of working-class identity. Here, I am following Mick Smith and Joyce Davidson (2008: 201) when they argue that 'gentrification reveals the presence of a dominant and dominating cultural ethos at work in urban transformations', a suggestion that I adhere to by showing that visions of retail regeneration privilege distinctively middle-class aesthetic and moral ideals.

Having established that this book is about the classed geographies of consumption, in Chap. 3, I begin to consider this relationship by describing some of the important shifts in the geographies of retail capital understood to have undermined the viability and vitality of many British High Streets. Here, a key threat to the High Street—alongside the rise of Internet shopping—has been the out-of-town retail park or Regional Shopping Centre. Since the 1980s, these spaces have been idealized as spaces of middle-class consumption, both domesticated and leisured. The privileged identity of such spaces as modern 'cathedrals' of consumption has cast a long shadow over the High Street, with juxtapositions of these seductive consumer landscapes with struggling High Streets feeding into narratives that equate the latter with social stigma and failure. As I explain in Chap. 4, this became a self-fulfilling prophecy, with the abandonment of shops on the High Street cementing the idea that these are dying and that those who use them are on the social and economic margins. It helps us understand why the rhetoric of those arguing for regeneration focuses on the need for *revitalization*, with the High Street being depicted as dead despite the fact it continues to play a key role in the economic and social life of British cities, especially for the urban poor.

Combined, Chaps. 3 and 4 show that discourses emphasizing the need for the transformation of the High Street support the wider logics of gentrification, an argument I clarify by showing how retail policy is encouraging the nascent gentrification of Margate. However, in the following chapters I move from considering general pronouncements about the health of the High Street to explore more specific policy debates and arguments against particular forms of retailing. These chapters emphasize that retail policy is not just classed, but also makes moral distinctions based on the age, gender and race of consumers. For example, in Chap. 5 I explore the policy debates that have raged around the nighttime city, and particularly the accusation that the High Street at night is given over to a form of youthful leisured consumption revolving around binge drinking and anti-social behaviour. Here, I show that policies intended to promote safer and more inclusive High Streets are encouraging a gentrification of nightlife that has obvious consequences for less affluent consumers, including residualized youth, working-class consumers and those from non-white ethnic minorities. In Chap. 6 I extend such perspectives on the remoralization of the High Street when I alight on controversies concerning the presence of sex shops, lap dance clubs and other 'sexualized' premises on the High Street, demonstrating that these betray anxieties about the decline of respectable femininities and masculinities in contemporary Britain. In Chap. 7, issues of class and gender are again to the fore, with the widespread representation of betting shops as places associated with residualized, dangerous masculinities supporting the argument that these need to be excised from the High Street.

Each of these examples shows that the arguments for High Street regeneration are replete with metaphors of disgust informed by classed stereotypes of class, race and gender. These moralizing discourses present an unanswerable case for action to be taken, and privilege an essentially nostalgic vision of the British High Street. In the latter sections of this book, I turn away from questions of blight and decline to consider specific elements of this vision, and the forms of consumption deemed appropriate on the British High Street. Chapter 8, for example, considers the rise of 'foodie-ism' on the High Street in the form of policies encouraging the conspicuous consumption of healthy, green and local food rather than fatty or fast food. While such policies can be understood unproblematically as attempts to improve health and well-being, I inject a note of caution by suggesting they support retail gentrification, and in some cases even contribute to poor health by closing down the options available to the less affluent, especially in areas understood to be multicultural. Chapter 9 develops themes of localism and authenticity by focusing on the way policies for High Streets intersect with 'artwashing' agendas promoting the creative economy. In this chapter, I argue that the promotion of High Streets as bohemian spaces can often promote a bourgeois agenda, and destroy the class diversity that might actually inspire creative and artistic endeavor. In a final chapter, I conclude that current policies for High Street regeneration, though persuasively presented and sometimes well-intentioned, are underpinned by visions of change that are ultimately exclusionary. Arguing against prescriptions promoting retail gentrification, the book ends by insisting on a more inclusive vision of the High Street, one recognizing the diverse forms of conviviality already present on many local shopping streets.

References

Bird, H. (2014). Betting shop power given to councils. *The Planner*, 30 April, http://www.theplanner.co.uk/news/betting-shop-planning-power-given-to-councils

British Retail Consortium (2009). *Twenty first century High Streets: A new vision for our town centres*. London: British Retail Consortium.

Bromley, R. D., & Matthews, D. L. (2007). Reducing consumer disadvantage: Reassessing access in the retail environment. *International Review of Retail, Distribution and Consumer Research, 17*(5), 483–501.

Bromley, R. D., & Thomas, C. T. (1995). Small town shopping decline: Dependence and inconvenience for the disadvantaged. *International Review of Retail, Distribution and Consumer Research, 5*(4), 433–456.

Carmona, M. (2014). London's local High Streets: The problems, potential and complexities of mixed street corridors. *Progress in Planning, 100*, 1–84.

Coca-Stefaniak, J. A. (2013). Successful town centres—Developing effective strategies. Gloucester, GFirst-ATCM, http://www.atcm.org/tools/successful-town-centres---developing-effective-strategies-.php

Cummins, S., & Macintyre, S. (1999). The location of food stores in urban areas: A case study in Glasgow. *British Food Journal, 101*(7), 545–553.

Davidson, M., & Wyly, E. (2012). Class-ifying London: Questioning social division and space claims in the post-industrial metropolis. *City, 16*(4), 395–421.

Department of Communities and Local Government (DCLG) (2012). *Reimagining urban spaces to revitalize our High Streets*. London: DCLG.

Digital High Street Advisory Board (2015). *Digital High Street 2020 Report*. London: Digital High Street Advisory Board.

Dorling, D., & Rees, P. H. (2003). A nation still dividing: The British census and social polarisation 1971–2001. *Environment and Planning A, 35*, 1287–1313.

External Advisory Group (2013). *National review of town centres: Community and enterprise in Scotland's town centres*. Edinburgh: Scottish Government.

Fenton, A., Lupton, R., Arrundale, R., & Tunstall, R. (2013). Public housing, commodification, and rights to the city: The US and England compared. *Cities, 35*, 373–378.

Ferreri, M. (2016). Pop-up shops as interruptions in (post-) recessional London. In J. Shirley and C. Lindner (eds) *Cities interrupted. Visual Culture and Urban Space.* London, Bloomsbury.

Findlay, A., & Sparks, L. (2009). *Literature review: Policies adopted to support a healthy retail sector and retail led regeneration and the impact of retail on the regeneration of town centres and local High Streets.* The Scottish Government: Edinburgh.

Georgiou, M. (2013). *Media and the city: Cosmopolitanism and difference.* Cambridge: Polity.

Gilson, J. (2014). Poundland and its ilk are an asset to today's High Streets. *The Guardian,* 20 February, http://www.theguardian.com/commentisfree/2014/feb/20/poundland-high-streets-betting-shops-pawnbrokers

Greater London Authority (2013). *Open for business: Empty shops on London's High Streets.* London: GLA.

Green, A., Autier, P., Boniol, M., Boyle, P., Dore, J. F., Gandini, S., et al. (2007). The association of use of sunbeds with cutaneous malignant melanoma and other skin cancers: A systematic review. *International Journal of Cancer, 120*(5), 1116–1122.

Grimsey, B. (2013) The Grimsey Review: An alternative future for the High Street. Retrieved from www.vanishinghighstreet.com

Guy, C. (1985). The food and grocery shopping behaviour of disadvantaged consumers: Some results from the Cardiff consumer panel. *Transactions of the Institute of British Geographers,* 181–190.

Guy, C., & David, G. (2004). Measuring physical access to 'healthy foods' in areas of social deprivation: A case study in Cardiff. *International Journal of Consumer Studies, 28*(3), 222–234.

Guy, C., Clarke, G., & Eyre, H. (2004). Food retail change and the growth of food deserts: A case study of Cardiff. *International Journal of Retail and Distribution Management, 32*(2), 72–88.

Hatherley, O. (2016). *The Ministry of Nostalgia.* London: Verso.

Hughes, C., & Jackson, C. (2015). Death of the High Street: Identification, prevention, reinvention. *Regional Studies, Regional Science, 2*(1), 236–255.

Jackson, P. (2016). Go Home Jamie: Reframing consumer choice. *Social & Cultural Geography.* doi:10.1080/14649365.2015.1124912.

Jones, O. (2012). *Chavs: The demonization of the working class.* London: Verso.

Kennell, J. (2011). Rediscovering cultural tourism: cultural regeneration in seaside towns. *Journal of Town & City Management, 1*(4), 364–380.

Labour Policy Review (2012). *Helping our High Streets: Empowering local communities.* London: Labour Party.

Le Grand, E. (2015) Linking moralization and class: The role of ressentiment and respectability in the social reaction to chavs. Sociological Research Online, 20(4), 15, http://www.socresonline.org.uk/20/4/15.html

Leventhal, T., & Brooks-Gunn, J. (2003). Moving to opportunity: An experimental study of neighborhood effects on mental health. *American Journal of Public Health, 93*(9), 1576–1582.

Lewis, B. (2013). High Streets thrive by community-led renewal (DCLG press release) https://www.gov.uk/government/news/high-streets-thrive-by-community-led-renewal

Leyshon, A., & Thrift, N. (1995). Geographies of financial exclusion: Financial abandonment in Britain and the United States. *Transactions of the Institute of British Geographers, 20*(3), 312–341.

Local Data Company (2015). *Vacancy rate Report H2 2015.* London: LDC.

Local Government Association (2012) LGA Survey—Strip clubs and bookies are hitting economic growth. LGA media release, 14 April 2012, http://www.local.gov.uk/media-centre/-/journal_content/56/10180/3376601/NEWS

Murray, C. D., & Turner, E. (2004). Health, risk and sunbed use: A qualitative study. *Health, Risk & Society, 6*(1), 67–80.

New Economics Foundation (2003). *Ghost town Britain: The threat from economic globalisation to livelihoods, liberty and local freedom.* London: NEF.

New Economics Foundation (2010). *Re-imagining the High Street: Escape from clone town Britain.* London: NEF.

Paget, A., & Birdwell, J. (2013). *Giving something back: Measuring the social value of charity shops.* London: Demos.

Portas, M. (2011). The Portas review: An independent review into the future of our High Streets. http://www.maryportas.com/news/2011/12/12/the-portas-review/

Portas, M. (2010). Supermarkets are killing local communities. The Daily Telegraph, 1 June, http://www.telegraph.co.uk/news/earth/agriculture/supermarkets/7791746/Mary-Portas-supermarkets-are-killing-local-communities.html

Portas, M. (2015). *Shop Girl: A memoir.* London: Doubleday.

Saner, E. (2011). Margate's miserable claim to fame. *The Guardian*, 18 February http://www.theguardian.com/business/2011/feb/18/margate-miserable-claim-to-fame

Schiller, R. (1986). Retail decentralisation: The coming of the third wave. *The Planner, 72*(7), 13–15.

Smith, M., & Davidson, J. (2008). Cities of etiquette and civility. In P. Hubbard, T. Hall, & J. R. Short (Eds.), *The Sage Companion to the City.* London: Sage.

Sparks, L. (1987). Retailing in enterprise zones: The example of Swansea. *Regional Studies, 21*(1), 37–42.

Speak, C. (2013). High Street blight: Are poundshops better than empty shops? The *Guardian*, 23 May, http://www.theguardian.com/uk/the-northerner/2013/may/23/high-street-blight-payday-lenders-pound-shops

Street-Porter, J. (2012). My Whitstable. *The Daily Telegraph*, 5 September, p. 23.

Swinney, P., & Sivaev, D. (2013). *Beyond the High Street: Why our city centres really matter*. London: Centre for Cities.

Taylor-Gooby, P., & Stoker, G. (2011). The coalition programme: A new vision for Britain or politics as usual? *The Political Quarterly, 82*(1), 4–15.

Townshend, T. G. (2016). Toxic High Streets. Journal of Urban Design, online early, doi:10.1080/13574809.2015.1106916

Watson, S., & Wells, K. (2005). Spaces of nostalgia: The hollowing out of a London market. *Social & Cultural Geography, 6*(1), 17–30.

Westlake, T., & Dagleish, K. (1990). Disadvantaged consumers—Can planning respond? *Planning Outlook, 33*(2), 118–123.

Westfield City. (2011). Press release: New Westfield city. Retrieved from http://uk.westfield.com/stratfordcity

Williams, P., & Hubbard, P. (2001). Who is disadvantaged? Retail change and social exclusion. *The International Review of Retail, Distribution and Consumer Research, 11*(3), 267–286.

Woodliffe, L. (2004). Rethinking consumer disadvantage: The importance of qualitative research. *International Journal of Retail & Distribution Management, 32*(11), 523–531.

Wrigley, N., & Brookes, E. (2015). The rise and effects of 'convenience culture'. In N. Wrigley & D. Lambiri (Eds.), *British High Streets: From crisis to recovery? A comprehensive review of the evidence*. Southampton: University of Southampton.

Wrigley, N., & Dolega, L. (2011). Resilience, fragility and adaptation: New evidence on the performance of UK High Streets during global economic crisis and its policy implications. *Environment and Planning A, 43*(10), 2337–2363.

Wrigley, N., Guy, C., & Lowe, M. (2002). Urban regeneration, social inclusion and large store development: The Seacroft development in context. *Urban Studies, 39*(11), 2101–2114.

Wrigley, N., Shaw, H., Lowe, M., Guy, C., & Wood, S. (2007). Relocalising food shopping. Consumer responses to supply chain transformation in the UK convenience store sector. Online verfügbar: www.nrpf.org/PDF/Relocalising_shopping.pdf

Young, I. M. (1990). The ideal of community and the politics of difference. In L. J. Nicholson (Ed.), *Feminism/Postmodernism*. New York: Routledge.

3

Going Out of Town

In many discourses of British retail decline, there's a palpable nostalgia for an imagined city in which community life revolved around the High Street. These, and town centres in general, are remembered as the focus of civic and cultural life, with retail spaces providing the stage on which encounters with others provided the 'social glue' that bonded communities together. This is an imagination arguably fuelled by our fascination with big city life, the density of urban living and the possibilities of metropolitan interaction (Dimendberg 2004). But in fact, it can be argued that in much of the twentieth century, the privileging of automobility prompted centrifugal rather than centripetal tendencies in British cities, with successive 'waves' of retail investment shifting the focus of community life firstly from the centre to the suburbs and latterly, to sites that were ex-urban, located on the periphery of cities or even on greenfield sites at some distance from the urban core (Schiller 1986). New landscapes of retail—the out-of-town superstore, the retail park, the out-of-town mall—ostensibly turned their back on the city, extolling the virtues of speed, immateriality and individual choice over traditional urban concepts of community, propinquity and shared sociality (Hubbard and Lilley 2004).

© The Editor(s) (if applicable) and The Author(s) 2017
P. Hubbard, *The Battle for the High Street*,
DOI 10.1057/978-1-137-52153-8_3

In this regard, the recent decline of the British High Street needs to be understood in the context of decades of retail decentralization, a move out of town that arguably decanted particular forms of consumption—and particular groups of consumers—away from town and city centres. As we have seen, there are certain dangers of exaggerating the impacts of out-of-town shopping, as clearly many of those who frequented peripheral sites also visited town centres (and vice versa). Not all of those who remained reliant on town centres could necessarily be described as disadvantaged consumers. But in terms of the imagined social and economic geography of British towns and cities, the impacts were unquestionably huge, with many High Streets appearing outdated and increasingly irrelevant long before the retail recession of the twenty-first century kicked in. In contrast, out-of-town sites appeared to offer a new form of shopping that was both profitable and popular, with their carefully cultivated atmosphere of leisured consumption at odds with the more spontaneous, intimate and even disordered forms of retailing traditional in town centre shops and street markets. And, above all else, it was the large, regional shopping centre of the 1980s and 1990s which was seen to have perfected this model of leisured consumption, fundamentally changing established ideas about how British retail landscapes reflect distinctions of class, space and place.

Scenes from a Mall

I was born a stone's throw from Bluewater, one of the UK's largest Regional Shopping Centres, growing up approximately five minutes' drive away on the Fleet Estate, a pleasant mixed development of semis, flats and maisonettes built by Dartford Town Council in collaboration with private developers in the 1960s. Except that when I lived there, the site of the future shopping centre was still a chalk pit owned by Blue Circle cement, something we were acutely aware of in the drought of 1976, when a patina of chalk dust thrown up by the lorries thundering down the nearby main road coated our parched lawns, waiting to be washed away by rains that never came. Moving away from Dartford in the late 1970s, I rarely gave another thought to the chalk pits, ignorant that they would occasionally double for some alien world in *Doctor Who*, with the production team evidently thinking a chalky wasteland on the periphery of South East London possessed suitably extra-terrestrial qualities.

By 1990, the chalk pits had long been worked out, and Blue Circle cement sought planning permission to develop the site. For a number of years, it looked like the site might go the way of many other local quarries—becoming a landfill site—until the Australian developers Land Lease became interested. Major retailers including *John Lewis*, *Marks and Spencers* and *Debenhams* were quickly brought on board, no doubt excited by the prospects of a site adjacent to the M25 London orbital motorway, and hence within an hours' drive time for millions of consumers in the affluent South East of England. The £375 million shopping centre opened in March 1999, one of the largest in Europe, providing nearly two million feet of sales space spread across a two-tier triangular mall.

Given I have often driven within a few miles of Bluewater, I have been to it surprisingly rarely. This given, once I have negotiated the queues that inevitably stack up on the approach road from the M25, the sight that greets me retains a certain capacity to shock. Nestling in the bottom of the quarry, surrounded by steep-sloped chalk cliffs and seven landscaped lakes, Bluewater looks nothing like a traditional shopping street, and more like a crashed alien spaceship, completely out of place, as if abandoned by the aforesaid *Doctor Who* special effects team; in his perambulation within the 'acoustic footprint' of the M25, psychogeographer Iain Sinclair invokes the Martian invaders of HG Wells' *War of the Worlds*. Going on, he ponders this Kentish spectacle and its capacity to draw in the metropolitan visitor:

> Pausing, in wonder, on the edge of the pit, I saw the weird beauty of this excavation. Virtual water, glass fountains, had replaced the tired Kentish shore as a place of pilgrimage. Bluewater is the new Margate. The sickly London child Samuel Palmer was sent to Thanet to convalesce; sea-bathing and sermons. T.S. Eliot nursed his soul-sickness at the Albermarle Hotel in Cliftonville. Such indulgences have been suspended: now perfectly healthy urbanites, pricked by subliminally induced desires, descend on Junction 2 of the M25. They follow the yellow signs to Bluewater. No need for further explanation, the name is enough. A retail paradise. No hassle. City of glass in a kaolin bowl. (Sinclair 2002: 5)

It's hard to disagree with his assessment of its uncanny appearance, and it's certainly a spectacle that has proved successful, with the Centre out-competing its rival Lakeside (eight miles away, in Essex) for customers in this part of estuary England. Land Lease boast on their website that over half a million visit the centre every week, and 72% are defined as 'ABC1', reflecting the fact that this is Britain's 'most affluent catchment', responsible for 10% of the annual retail spend in Britain.

At ground level, Bluewater presents a less-impressive façade, the tarmac expanses of the car parks culminating in entrances that are far from obvious, and architecturally undistinguished in any way. Inside, the centre lacks real focal points and the type of grand ensemble theatrics that characterized some of the progenitors of Bluewater (like the now-defunct monorail at Merry Hill, Dudley, or the themed indoor fairground at the Metro Centre, Gateshead). In his indictment of the design mediocrity characterizing austerity Britain, Owen Hatherley (2012: 29) seizes upon Bluewater as paradigmatic. Puzzling over how the shopping centre is even accessible by foot (answer: it is not), he is surprised by its internal architectural blandness—repetitive urban forms, unmemorable motifs, materials that soothe, but do not jar, and subdued public art and public seating in abundance—but also comments on the sheer spectacle it provides with 'thousands of people browsing, watching, buying, eating or expelling their waste', something he finds 'thrilling, in its way'. The beauty of appearance is then trumped by the beauty of interactivity, with 'hyperaesthetic hedonism' celebrated in a normative architectural form that breaks down traditional divides between private and public, inside and outside (Philippopoulos-Mihalopoulos 2014).

This combination of the inoffensive architecture and the display of consumer ritual—shopping as leisure, leisure as shopping—has been described as symptomatic of contemporary consumer society. The blandness of form, and the lack of real place identity, is viewed as intentional, the consequence of developers constructing an environment in which global brands and global shoppers are interchangeable. There's nothing too quirky, or characterful, here given a mall in Dartford, Kent has to work in the same manner as a mall pretty much anywhere else in the world. The mall then is a classic example of what anthropologist Marc Augé (1995) terms a 'non-place': a place lacking a history, or geography, as the individual has only one reason to be in that space (consumption) and the overall intention is to produce similitude, not difference. But allusions to globality are never total. Indeed, Bluewater is a space where some local place referents are admitted, such as the 'Thames Walk' *bas relief* on the lower levels of the mall. But these attempts to inject a little local character are not allowed to distract from the familiar signs and symbols of the global consumer brandscape. The 330 or so shops present themselves in the same way that they might do in a retail mall in Shanghai, Sydney or San Francisco. Brand names in the window, cool façades, ordered, subdued. No ad hoc retailing or bargain bins piled on the pavements here, the stores know their place and aim to draw the consumer in, not impose upon them.

This polite mode of address is at the heart of the shopping experience at Bluewater. When I make my journey there, I am in search of a coat, which ultimately involves a circumnavigation of the entire mall given the three big Department Stores are located as anchors at the vertices of its triangular form. But the journey round, despite the crowds, is relatively smooth. I do not have to navigate traffic, save the odd mobility scooter, and I am not interrupted by the Big Issue sellers, charity workers and miscellaneous 'data muggers' that I would anticipate meeting if out shopping on the average High Street. The travel, like the floor, is smooth, and while it's not entirely clear how the affective cues of surfaces, light and feel are designed into the spaces in ways that encourage particular directions of movement, it's hard to resist a journey that does not take in all three sides of the centre. No doubt, given the way architectural devices are integrated into contemporary buildings to influence movement (Bissell 2009), careful thought was given to such issues and the engineering of flow.

However, this achievement of circulation—the flow of consuming bodies—is not just an outcome of self-regulation and architectural persuasion. There's also surveillance. When I visit the Centre I am only dimly aware of security guards, or the army of those who clean and maintain the Centre. But knowing that this is the Shopping Centre notorious for banning the wearing of hooded tops in 2005, targeting the teenage trend of the time (much to the disgust of youth charities), I was keeping a keen eye out for some of the reputed 350 CCTV cameras which Iain Sinclair (2002: 6) suggests pour images onto digital tapes 'that chart drugged shoppers leaving ectoplasmic contrails'. The aim of surveillance is, of course, to protect the visiting public and clamp down on any anti-social behaviour that might create alarm or distress, but there's an extensive literature alleging that this type of surveillance is routinely used to scrutinize—and exclude—those who simply appear to be in the mall for purposes other than leisured consumption. These 'non-consumers' might include the homeless or itinerant populations who regard malls as a source of food and shelter, political activists or protestors seeking to promote ethical consumption, or simply those teenage 'mall rats' who hang out without necessarily spending very much. Despite allegations of discrimination on the basis of gender and ethnicity (see Norris and Armstrong 1999), shopping centre managers typically justify this scrutiny with reference to producing a 'family-friendly' environment: in relation to the aforementioned hoodie ban, Bluewater's property manager Helen Smith went on public record to state 'We're very concerned that some of our guests don't feel at all comfortable in what really is a family environment'.

Bluewater in many ways conforms to Malcolm Voyce's (2006: 26) view that the contemporary shopping mall is like a 'prison in reverse': the aim is to keep deviant behaviour on the outside and maintain a consumerist ambience inside. But is not just non-conforming behaviour that is kept outside. Danny Miller et al. (1998) note that the out-of-town mall reproduces culture/nature distinctions by excluding all but the most tamed of natures: plants, animals, and even the weather are excluded in the interests of creating a civil, constantly unchanging and predictable shopping environment. This exclusion, by and large, goes unnoticed and uncommented upon, to the extent that when a deer wandered into a shopping centre in Norwich, or a fox was spotted near the bins at the back of Surrey Quays shopping centre, it became the subject of news headlines. Bluewater too feels hermetically sealed, outside both space and time, keeping the imagined terrors of the outside world at bay. On my visit there I barely register the passing of time, and the bright, pleasant interior makes me forget the persistent grey mizzle outside. Even the thermal environment is controlled, inducing an affective state among shoppers making them more susceptible to enticements to purchase (Healy 2014).

For critical urbanists, Bluewater, and other highly engineered retail spaces, have been of concern as they symbolize an undemocratic urban form that feigns welcome to all, but which actually offers little flexibility or freedom. They are, as Rob Shields (1989) has argued, single-minded spaces, despite the efforts designers go to in an attempt to manufacture the illusion that something else other than mere shopping is going on. The mall is then a pseudo-space that works through spatial strategies of 'dissemblance and duplicity' (Shields 1989: 151). For example, the branding of malls as 'family spaces' is inherently misleading, a shorthand suggesting a playful space in which children and the elderly are equally welcome, whereas, in reality, the mall is defined around middle-aged adultist norms. Indeed, the types of 'anti-social behavior' discouraged by some malls are often much more social than shopping is, but viewed through the eyes of middle-aged consumers, young people sitting around in groups chatting, laughing and flirting are using the mall for a purpose other than that considered 'normal'. Elaborating, Joyce Davidson and Mick Smith (2007) have suggested that the real crime of young people hanging out in shopping centres is not that they do not consume at all (after all, the malls sell the hoodies they wear), but they consume in the wrong way, embodying a particular set of norms that are simply 'out of place'. Shields (1989: 160) concludes that, for young people to fit in, they must 'observe bourgeois forms and modes of social docility, and a conservatism in both dress and action'. For children's geographers like Hugh Matthews et al. (2000), this is a matter of deep regret, for in an era where young people are increasingly regarded with suspicion when encountered in public space unaccompanied by adults, the mall provides a warm and safe 'third space' for young people between school and home.

In this sense, 'family values' are actually middle-class values, with the desire of mall developers being to create an ambience of leisured consumption undisturbed by the incursion of those who are not prepared to consume in the desired manner. Putting it bluntly, Goss (1993: 24) argues that 'the shopping centre is a strongly bounded or purified social space that excludes a significant minority of the population … Malls are spaces for white middle classes'. The implication here is that shopping centres such as Bluewater 'filter the middle classes away from unnecessary social influences and interruptions to the intensity of their spending' (Voyce 2006: 27), and, as such, offer a sanitized version of the shopping experience one might experience on the High Street. Indeed, as I move around Bluewater, there are none of the signs of poverty, vandalism or abandonment that I might expect to find on the nearby High Streets of Dartford and Gravesend, which have among the highest vacancy rates of any High Street in the South East. All of the shops appear to be let, and more or less everybody who is not working here appears to be consuming in some form or other. But the mall does appear to be quite diverse in terms of its users, who are far from all white English, with a range of accents and languages suggesting a cosmopolitan constituency drawn from different areas of London, and not just the whiter commuter dormitories of Kent, Sussex and Surrey. Not all are splurging on designer goods either, with many clutching single carrier bags indicating they have been purchasing discount sportswear or something from *Debenhams*' 'Blue Cross' sale. Some do not appear to have bought anything at all. And even though it's a school day, I notice a few teenagers walking around with friends, and nobody is challenging their right to be there. Perhaps then we need to be more open to the idea that these spaces do have a certain 'looseness', and even if they can never be truly part of the public sphere, provide some of the qualities of social mixing that we more routinely associate with town centres and High Streets (see also Georgiou 2013; Parlette and Cowen 2011).

Distinction, Space and Place

Bluewater is not a typical British mall, given that the majority of these were actually developed in-town in the 1960s and 1970s by British companies (most notably the Arndale Property Trust), some featuring indoor markets and stores owned by independent traders. But the emergence of Bluewater, and the new generation of out-of-town malls—Sheffield's Meadowhall, Merry Hill in the Black Country, Gateshead's Metro Centre, Cribbs Causeway (outside Bristol), Essex's Lakeside—certainly seemed to signal a fundamental shift in the nature of retailing in the UK in the last decades of the twentieth century. 'Shopping-centre capitalism' (Crewe 2008) became the subject of considerable academic debate, with many connecting the rise of the Regional Shopping Centre to both the *laissez faire* planning regime introduced by the Thatcher governments and the wider cultural legacy of the 1980s. However, some retail geographers and cultural theorists stepped further back, seeing the rise of the Regional Shopping Centre as indicative of a more fundamental shift in the nature of global society, one that went far beyond the machinations of the British government and the loosening of planning controls. The narrative here was one in which the decline of the industrial base of much of the urbanized West, and associated shifts in the global economy, was deemed to have ushered in a 'consumer society'. This thesis suggested that consumption had become the driving force behind the economy, with consumption no longer the reward for work but the main form of work. Consumption intensified and diversified to encompass all facets of social life, with the transition from industrialism to post-industrialism requiring the rise of the *reflexive consumer*. This was—and is—a consumer adept at reordering the signs and symbols of everyday life in the search for identity (Clarke and Bradford 1998), a consumer for whom acts of consumption went well beyond the purchase of traditional goods and services, being imbricated in a process of constructing a 'lifestyle'. The use of a good or commodity began to be subordinated to its symbolic value, with image becoming profoundly important (Fig. 3.1). The most mundane of commodities began to be sold as objects of desire, with design, image and affect saturating consumption (Gabriel and Lang 2008).

Many studies of reflexive consumption hence emphasized the connection between 'post-modernism' and the rise of a consumer society. For example, the notion of 'lifestyle shopping' described by Rob Shields (1992) was explicitly informed by ideas about the importance of identity in postmodern society. Postmodernism, associated with the breakdown of the 'cultural logic' of the modern industrial era, was characterized as representing a crisis of science, progress, and metanarrative and a consequent prioritization of complexity, contingency, and plurality. It happened in the context of new understandings of risk. New global challenges—climate change, pandemic, terrorism—underscored the fact that the modern state was no longer capable of generating the 'ontological security' subjects desired (Beck 1992). In fact, science and industry became seen as a source of risk, not the means of avoiding it. Consequently, Shields suggested that people sought the sense of belonging and certainty that was once provided by the state and paid work through individual (and often creative) acts of consumption. Identifying the importance of aestheticized

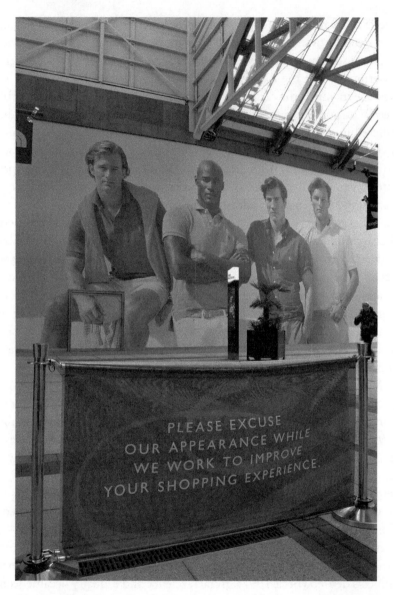

Fig. 3.1 Keeping up appearances at the mall: Gunwharf Quays Designer Shopping Outlet, Portsmouth (photo: author)

consumption as a means of self-actualization, differentiation, and distinction, Shields thus echoed Jean Baudrillard's (1970) arguments about the triumph of symbolic overuse or exchange values when he argued 'shopping for goods is a social activity built around social exchange as well as simple commodity exchange' (Shields 1992: 16). In the consumer society, the consumption of goods and services may well be about assuaging needs, but it has been stressed that those needs were being shaped by a symbolic economy that had long lost any obvious relationship to the human costs of production.

Developing these ideas about identity and consumption, Zygmunt Bauman provided an influential theorization of the role of consumption in instigating a logic of social control based not so much on state surveillance, but on the relentlessly individualized pursuit of identity and surety through acts of consumption:

> The distinctive mark of the consumer society and its consumerist culture is not...consumption as such; not even the elevated and fast-rising volume of consumption. What sets the members of consumer society apart from their ancestors is the emancipation of consumption from its past instrumentality that used to draw its limits—the demise of 'norms' and the new plasticity of 'needs', setting consumption free from functional bonds and absolving it from the need to justify itself with reference to anything but its own pleasurability. (Bauman 2000: 12–13)

Suggesting individuals are destined to seek 'biographical solutions to systemic contradictions in the marketplace', Bauman spells out the self-perpetuating logic of the consumer society: 'to become a consumer means to be dependent for one's survival. .. on the consumer market' (Bauman 2001: 25). Desires are never fulfilled, as they are not based on any notion of need except the perceived need for distinction and difference. The manipulation of meaning in the marketplace ensures this desire is fuelled by desire. The consumer is condemned to continue consuming, as distinction can never be fully achieved, with the constant reinvention of self, required in the context of changing cultural norms and values.

In effect, the new theories concerning the rise of consumer society suggested that the rigid class-based identities of industrial society (based on one's position in relation to the means of production) were being super-seded by social identities based on consumption. These were arguably more fluid, and less fixed, than had been the case in the past, constructed through the purchase of goods offering the promise of a ready-made 'lifestyle'. But does this mean that class has disappeared in a mélange of signs and symbols? To the contrary, sociologists argued class has persisted, but not in the strictly stratified sense it was previously understood. For Bev Skeggs (2015), class is inherently about consumption, but the ability to consume, display and 'own' culture is not evenly distributed. Consumer goods and lifestyles are the status markers mapped onto class relations, but some evidently lack the resources to consume 'properly' and hence are unable to show their lives have 'value'. For example, some middle-class commentators routinely mock the working class for their consumption behaviour, and reduce this to a question of lifestyle choices rather than seeing this as constrained by material circumstances. The working classes, we are told, shop at *Primark* and other discount clothes stores, despite their reputation for importing 'sweat shop' garments, because they are ignorant of the ethics of 'fair trade' consumption; they eat at *McDonalds* despite the damage mass-produced beef does to the environment; they drink cheap, high alcohol ciders and flavoured vodkas because they want to get drunk quickly; and they gamble away much of the little money they have. In short, they fail to act as ethical, knowledgeable consumers. It's hardly surprising those populations described as exhibiting working-class consumption habits typically dis-identify with such classification because they feel it represents them as 'excessive, fecund, irresponsible and pathological' (Skeggs 2015: 217). It's this that can encourage indebtedness, with the individuals that can least afford it sometimes 'splashing out' on designer goods that show they too have 'taste' (something equally mocked by middle classes, who see this form of conspicuous consumption as vulgar and ostentatious).

The consumer society is then one where inequality abounds, with shopping being an arena where there's a constant struggle over who—and what—is valued. Pierre Bourdieu's (1984) classic survey of the relations of class and taste remains important here, given that it shows that differences in taste or aesthetic preference are far from incidental in class struggles, with distinctions of class being associated with the construction of complex 'regimes of taste'. Recognizing that not everyone can participate in this struggle on equal terms, Bauman (2000) develops

Bourdieu's thesis by speaking of the existence of *tourists* and *vagabonds*. While the former describes a seduced consumer on an endless journey of consumption made with the aim of expressing and maintaining distinction, the latter is the term Bauman uses to describe those repressed populations on the margins of consumer society, endlessly journeying from place to place because they are unwelcome in many retail and leisure spaces. These are the populations unable (or unwilling) to participate in the rituals of tasteful, leisured consumption, flawed others whose lifestyles are devalued, and judged unsuitable for commodification. So while there's an ongoing struggle for status and distinction within the middle classes, there's an often violent intolerance expressed towards those who reside outside the mainstream of consumer society, those who cannot afford to fully participate because of poverty or bad debt, those who are morally and culturally condemned for a poverty that is 'deserved' (Tyler 2015).

Developing such ideas about distinction, urban scholars have suggested there's a mutual fit between the vicissitudes of consumer society and the contemporary landscape of Western cities, with the search for new certainties through acts of consumption having an obvious spatial corollary in the proliferation of new spaces of retail such as the mall, but also the themed arcade, dockside outlet centre or luxury fashion district (see Goss 1993; Crewe 2015). All are spatially and socially distinct from the 'traditional' High Street and are not just settings for the sale of goods, being best thought of as resources on which consumers draw in their search for distinction. In such settings, the 'process of consumption accordingly starts before the actual purchase of the product' (Miles 2010: 2), since 'the spaces and places in which consumption occurs are as important as the products and services consumed' (Craik 1997: 125). This is not necessarily a new phenomenon, as historians have described some of the earliest sites of 'modern consumption'—such as the nineteenth-century department store, or arcade—as sites where the middle classes could display their fashions and taste free from the intrusion of the working classes. But in contemporary consumer society, the dictum 'you are where you shop' appears more fitting than ever, with shops and businesses positioning themselves within ever-changing hierarchies of taste through subtle aesthetic gestures and attempts to engineer a particular ambience. The decision to buy one's food in *Lidl* rather than *Waitrose*, for example, is one not solely determined by price, but is connected to store layout, the presentation of goods, and the way both stores avail upon the streetscape.

The aesthetics and design of space are then vital for framing acts of consumption, creating a saturated symbolic landscape that provokes particular associative moods and dispositions in the shopper by putting certain taste cultures 'on display'. As we have seen at Bluewater, motifs and designs can be carefully arrayed to create an experience that takes the consumer away from the here-and-now, creating the sense that something other than simply shopping is occurring. By combining 'carnival, festival and tourism in a single, total environment' (Goss 1993: 28), a sense of liminality is created, and though shopping is often a nerve-shattering and foot-blistering experience, the mall has been dominantly narrated as a space of leisure, a dream world which blurs representation and reality, time and space. In the 1980s and 1990s in particular, to shop in an out-of-town Regional Shopping Centre was to mark one's self off as displaying distinction and privilege, to show an appreciation of the new and the fashionable. At the same time, it was a potent way to display a sense of distaste towards the working-class cultures that were more routinely displayed on the High Street—a less contrived, and hence more disordered, space.

But synergies between leisure and retailing arguably went deeper. As retail capital gravitated to out-of-town and edge city locations to capture the spending of the mobile middle classes, the leisure industries surely followed, altering long-established patterns of 'going out' (Hubbard 2002). The multiplex cinema was incorporated into many Regional Shopping Centres, or became the focus of out-of-town Family Entertainment Complexes where it thrived alongside pizza restaurants and ten-pin bowling. Some commentators lamented the decline of the High Street as the predominant site of leisured consumption, and mourned the closure of town centre cinemas, theatres, bowling alleys and ice rinks. By and large, the shift to out-of-town was welcomed, with new sites of leisure readily incorporated into the lives and lifestyles of the mobile middle classes (Hubbard 2002). But given that they effaced much of the diversity and spontaneity of urban life in favour of a more predictable ambience, the result of such moves out of town was the creation of a more standardized consumption package which reduced the specificity of urban identity (Zukin 1998). Out-of-town leisure parks, retail parks and Regional Shopping Centres deployed similar logics, offering spaces of consumption easily accessible by car, comfortable, leisurely and thoroughly mediated. Simultaneously, they aimed to protect consumers from the 'moral confusion' that might arise from a confrontation with social difference (Jayne 2005), being spaces free from any social 'contamination'. In contrast, the High Street—long understood as a thoroughly modern space for displays of taste and style (Glennie and Thrift 1992)—had begun to appear thoroughly workaday, and even outdated, an environment associated with 'distress' purchases borne out of necessity, not a place the discerning would choose to visit. Descriptions of High Streets as dirty and dangerous began to abound. As we have seen, they began to be described as serving a fundamentally different type of consumer than out-of-town malls, being depicted overwhelmingly as spaces of flawed, working-class consumption.

High Streets Rediscovered?

The emergence of mediatized, privatized, serially reproduced consumer spaces on the periphery of many British towns and cities in the 1980s and 1990s represented a significant challenge to the dominance of the High Street as a site for retail and leisure spending. The potential threat to the High Street was consequently noted, with the observation that much of the vibrancy and vitality was being sucked out of the town centres neighbouring the Regional Shopping Centres, ringing alarm bells. Indeed, it was the plight of High Streets in towns like Dudley (near Merry Hill) or Rotherham (near Meadowhall) that initiated government policies discouraging the further development of out-of-town shopping centres, a reaction that has had some impact. Since the opening of the Trafford Centre near Manchester in 1998, and Bluewater in 1999, there have been few retail schemes that have come anywhere near these in size and scale. Those that have (e.g. the Westfield shopping centre in East London, West Quay in Southampton or Highpoint in Leicester) are in town, and more integrated within existing public transport networks, meaning they are theoretically more accessible to the car-less consumer (Lowe 2005). The out-of-town shopping centre, in effect, moved back to the city.

But irrespective of this putative return of retail capital to the city, the die had been cast, with the Regional Shopping Centre creating new standards and expectations amongst middle-class shoppers who had come to regard shopping as a form of leisure. For many, the shopping trip itself had become 'important than the actual purchase' (Miles 2010: 100). New in-town centres like Westfield, Stratford City, consequently market themselves as event destinations. As Rob Hollands and Paul Chatterton (2003) note, such in-town consumer spaces mimic out-of-town malls by targeting the mobile and wealthy, albeit they arguably market themselves most aggressively to young professional service workers and 'trendy' urbanites. But, just like the Regional Shopping Centre, they are not necessarily welcoming to younger teens, the homeless, the poor or the elderly. Anna Minton—author of *Ground Control: fear and happiness in the twenty-first century city*—highlights as much when she narrates Westfield Stratford City as part of the ongoing privatization of London, and implicated in an ongoing class polarization:

> My negative view stems from the sharp, visible polarization. Take the Westfield shopping centre in Stratford City—you don't even have to know you are in Stratford. You've come by tube or you've come straight in by motorway, which has taken you to the car park. You can go shopping. But if you make the effort to look across the road from the top of the entrance staircase, and you look down over the gyratory system, you've got this run-down 1970s mall, which is where many local people go. I think that really sharp social segregation in the city is unhealthy. (Minton 2014: 35)

Indeed, while the Westfield shopping centre looks, at first glance, to be used by a cross-section of the British population (Georgiou 2013, describing it as thoroughly cosmopolitan), it is, like Bluewater, predominantly marketed at the AB demographic, with the more affordable range of eateries and stores around its ground level food court (*Primark, Spud U Like, Greggs*) giving way to glossier global brands on the upper levels: *Karen Millen, Hugo Boss, Armani, Lacoste* (Fig. 3.2). Across the street, the 1970s-built Stratford Centre is a different proposition, with its vacant units, independent jewelers, mobile phone shops and discount indoor market drawing parallels with High Streets like Dudley and Dartford that live in the shadow of a Regional Shopping Centre. And the parallels do not end there, as while Stratford Westfield City is assiduously patrolled and surveyed, teenagers congregate around the Stratford Centre every night to skate and rollerblade, their presence allegedly tolerated in the interests of keeping them away from the more upscale mall across the way.

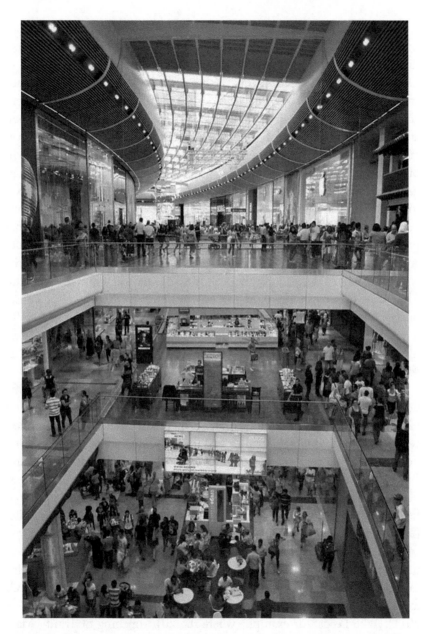

Fig. 3.2 The modern agora: Stratford Westfield Shopping Centre (photo: Sirje S. Flickr, used under a CC-BY license)

This type of analysis supports the idea that there's a continuing relationship between contemporary consumer culture and the creation of a more divided city (Dorling and Rees 2003). This is something emphasized in descriptions of two-speed or 'dual' cities, urban space being characteristically divided between the neighbourhoods associated with a mobile, affluent consumer class and the devalued, apparently dangerous, spaces of the less affluent—'wild zones' which the rich and powerful pass through or over as fast as possible (Urry 2004). Even if this does not neatly map onto an in-town/out-of-town divide, consideration of patterns of recent retail investment suggests a significant switch away from traditional, multi-use shopping streets towards essentially enclosed and privatized consumer spaces. Therefore, while in past epochs, Western cities were characterized by urban development that provided 'social richness' through the construction of parks, squares, avenues and open monuments (Lefebvre 2004: 52), in the contemporary city the enclosed mall or dockside outlet stands as the paradigmatic urban form. These sites present shopping as the 'only solution to the traumatic consequences of a failed modernity and a failed industrialisation' (Miles 2010: 10), seducing the middle class with a promise of escapism and opportunity, devaluing the industrial city of yesteryear—and 'distasteful' forms of working-class consumption—by turning their back on traditional retail environments.

But there are contradictions here, for, as more and more spaces become devoted to upmarket consumption, and the mall proliferates both in and out of town, the urge for differentiation increases. After all, consumption is strongly oriented around brands and identities that are available internationally, meaning retail brandscapes can easily become blandscapes (Bell and Binnie 2005). Middle-class consumers are, as Gabriel and Lang (2006) stress, fickle and unmanageable, gravitating towards new retail sites in the search for distinction as the older ones begin to lose their lustre. As Steven Miles (2010) notes, consumption spaces work by offering a sense of expanse to the consumer in which they feel they are having a different kind of experience to the norm. When this sense of escape or liminality fades, and the mall begins to appear normal, or even mundane, the mobile consumer begins a search for another consumer space. Even malls die over time (Parlette and Cowen 2011). Take Leeds, for example, where the 2013 opening of Trinity Mall, boasting 120 outlets including multiple 'pop-up' eateries, replaced the 1970s Leeds Shopping Plaza on the same site, with the Merrion Centre (originally built in 1964) to the north now looking decidedly threadbare and cheap in comparison to the newer additions to the city's retail offer. But even some of the retailers in the new mall have already moved on, and in 2014, a new Victoria Gate shopping centre, anchored by *John Lewis*, was announced, constructed around a spectacular, late nineteenth century glass-roofed arcade.

This ongoing search for distinction, and the spectre of obsolescence and unprofitability that this raises, means that local character and vernacular style are often seized upon by developers as retail capital seeks new, more profitable sites for its own realization. As the literatures on retail gentrification demonstrates, it's here that even previously marginalized inner city districts and High Streets can be fair game (Lloyd 2002): offbeat elements of street culture can be co-opted as deprived neighbourhoods become gradually incorporated in the middle-class cognitive map, each discoursed as a vibrant and vital part of the consumer city. These neighbourhoods become places, bequeathing cultural capital on the 'knowing' consumer prepared to step outside the mainstream, to experience something more local and 'authentic' than the retail offer elsewhere. The first sign of gentrification is typically the emergence of edgy art galleries, boutiques and trendy eateries, 'pop-up' outlets that quickly become known as the haunt of knowing 'hipsters'. But, as Ico Maly and Piia Varis (2015) point out, hipster culture is *translocal*, and the search for distinction via authenticity shares certain characteristics whether in the USA, Germany, or the UK (with the consumption of real coffee, vintage clothes, craft beer, and indie music appearing indexical). In the process, through interactions with hipster consumers from elsewhere, and increasing mediation, these neighbourhoods become gradually incorporated into global consumer cultures, even if a residuum of local culture survives (Zukin and Kosta 2004). Indeed, 'local character' is a globally recognizable package, but it's not one necessarily associated with immigrant or ethnic shopping per se (Hall 2012). Instead, it's something defined by a loose coalition of retail entrepreneurs, local government officials, media commentators, residents and incomers seeking to discourse a given shopping street as on-trend, uber-cool and authentic (Zukin 2011).

It's in this light that we must understand the threatened gentrification of High Streets in Britain as related to wider processes of retail restructuring in a consumer era, and an ongoing search for distinction on behalf of the middle classes. While the mall is a space of seduction, and a defensive setting in which 'unruly' working-class consumption is regarded as a sign of deviance, it appears that its hermetic nature has ultimately encouraged some middle-class consumers to venture back to the High Street in the search for something more real, and more distinctive. For some, the mall is perhaps just too self-contained, too brand-dominated. More traditional shopping streets, though widely regarded as more 'risky', gritty and even crime-ridden than the mall, can, it seems, sometimes be re-imagined as lively, hip and happening, attracting back the middle-class shoppers that abandoned the High Street for the mall in previous decades. Young hip urbanites are particularly courted, their aesthetic discrimination recognized via attempts to create a freewheeling bohemian vibe. As we will see, this often entails a gradual infiltration of the existing local retail scene by new alliances of class and capital. However, at times, it also entails less subtle forms of symbolic violence, and an outright condemnation of the working class, their tastes and ways of life.

References

Augé, M. (1995). *Non-place*. London: Verso.

Baudrillard, J. (1970). *The consumer society: Myths and structures*. Lodnon: Sage.

Bauman, Z. (2000). Urban battlefields of time/space wars. *Politologiske Studier* 7 (September), http://www.politologiske.dk/artikel01-ps7.htm

Bauman, Z. (2001). Consuming life. *Journal of Consumer Culture, 1*(1), 9–29.

Beck, U. (1992). *Risk Society*. London: Sage.

Bell, D., & Binnie, J. (2005). What's eating Manchester? Gastro-culture and urban regeneration. *Architectural Design, 75*(3), 78–85.

Bissell, D. (2009). Conceptualising differently-mobile passengers: Geographies of everyday encumbrance in the railway station. *Social & Cultural Geography, 10*(2), 173–195.

Bourdieu, P. (1984). *Distinction: A social critique of the judgment of taste*. Cambridge: Harvard University Press.

Chatterton, P., & Hollands, R. (2003). *Urban nightscapes: Youth cultures, pleasure spaces and corporate power*. London: Routledge.

Clarke, D. B., & Bradford, M. G. (1998). Public and private consumption and the city. *Urban Studies, 35*(5/6), 865–883.

Craik, J. (1997). The culture of tourism: Transformations of travel and theory. In C. Rojek & J. Urry (Eds.), *Touring cultures*. London: Routlege.

Crewe, L. (2008). Ugly beautiful? Counting the cost of the global fashion industry. *Geography, 93*(1), 25.

Crewe, L. (2015). Placing fashion: Art, space, display and the building of luxury fashion markets through retail design. Progress in Human Geography, online early, doi: 10.1177/0309132515580815

Dimendberg, E. (2004). Film noir and the spaces of modernity. Cambridge MA: Harvard University Press.

Dorling, D., & Rees, P. H. (2003). A nation still dividing: The British census and social polarisation 1971–2001. Environment and Planning A, 35, 1287–1313.

Gabriel, Y., & Lang, T. (2006). The unmanageable consumer. London: Sage.

Gabriel, Y., & Lang, T. (2008). New faces and new masks of today's consumer. Journal of Consumer Culture, 8(3), 321–340.

Georgiou, M. (2013). Media and the city: Cosmopolitanism and difference. Cambridge: Polity.

Glennie, P. D., & Thrift, N. J. (1992). Modernity, urbanism, and modern consumption. Environment and Planning D: Society and Space, 10(4), 423–443.

Goss, J. (1993). The "Magic of the Mall": An analysis of form, function, and meaning in the contemporary retail built environment. Annals of the Association of American Geographers, 83(1), 18–47.

Hall, S. M. (2012). City, street and citizen: The measure of the ordinary. London: Routledge.

Hatherley, O. (2012). A new kind of bleak: Journeys through urban Britain. London: Verso.

Healy, S. (2014). Atmospheres of consumption: Shopping as involuntary vulnerability. Emotion, Space and Society, 10, 35–43.

Hubbard, P. (2002). Screen-shifting consumption, 'riskless risks' and the changing geographies of cinema. Environment and Planning A, 34(7), 1239–1258.

Hubbard, P., & Lilley, K. (2004). Pacemaking the modern city: The urban politics of speed and slowness. Environment and Planning D: Society and Space, 22(2), 273–294.

Jayne, M. (2005). Cities and consumption. London: Routledge.

Lefebvre, H. (2004). Rhythmanalysis: Space, time and everyday life. London: Continuum.

Lloyd, R. (2002). Neo–bohemia: Art and neighborhood redevelopment in Chicago. Journal of Urban Affairs, 24(5), 517–532.

Lowe, M. (2005). The regional shopping centre in the inner city: A study of retail-led urban regeneration. Urban Studies, 42(3), 449–470.

Maly, I. & Varis, P. (2015). The 21st-century hipster: On micro-populations in times of superdiversity. European Journal of Cultural Studies, online early, doi:1367549415597920

Matthews, H., Taylor, M., Percy-Smith, B., & Limb, M. (2000). The unacceptable flaneur: The shopping mall as a teenage hangout. Childhood, 7(3), 279–294.

Miles, S. (2010). *Spaces for consumption*. London: Sage.

Miller, D., Jackson, P., Thrift, N., Holbrook, B., & Rowlands, M. (1998). *Shopping, place, and identity*. London: Routledge.

Minton, A. (2014). A conversation with Anna Minton. In R. Imrie & L. Lees (Eds.), *Sustainable London? The future of a global city*. Bristol: Policy Press.

Norris, C., & Armstrong, G. (1999). *The maximum surveillance society: The rise of CCTV*. Oxford: Berg.

Parlette, V., & Cowen, D. (2011). Dead malls: Suburban activism, local spaces, global logistics. *International Journal of Urban and Regional Research, 35*(4), 794–811.

Philippopoulos-Mihalopoulos, A. (2014). *Spatial justice: Body, lawscape, atmosphere*. London: Routledge.

Schiller, R. (1986). Retail decentralisation: The coming of the third wave. *The Planner, 72*(7), 13–15.

Shields, R. (1989). Social spatialisation and the built environment: The case of the West Edmonton Mall. *Environment and Planning D: Society and Space, 7*(2), 147–164.

Shields, R. (Ed.) (1992). *Lifestyle shopping: The subject of consumption*. Routledge: London.

Sinclair, I. (2002). At Bluewater. *London Review of Books*, 3 January, p. 5–7.

Skeggs, B. (2015). Introduction: Stratification or exploitation, domination, dispossession and devaluation? *The Sociological Review, 63*(2), 205–222.

Smith, C. (2007). *One for the girls!: The pleasures and practices of reading women's porn*. London: Intellect Books.

Tyler, I. (2015). Classificatory struggles: Class, culture and inequality in neoliberal times. *The Sociological Review, 63*(2), 493–511.

Urry, J. (2004). The 'system' of automobility. *Theory, Culture & Society, 21*(4-5), 25–39.

Voyce, M. (2006). Shopping malls in Australia: The end of public space and the rise of "consumerist citizenship"? *Journal of Sociology, 42*(3), 269–286.

Zukin, S. (1998). Urban lifestyles: Diversity and standardisation in spaces of consumption. *Urban Studies, 35*(5–6), 825–839.

Zukin, S. (2011). *Naked city the death and life of authentic urban places*. Oxford: Oxford University Press.

Zukin, S., & Kosta, E. (2004). Bourdieu off-Broadway: Managing distinction on a shopping block in the East Village. *City & Community, 3*(2), 101–114.

4

Reviving the High Street

Since the onset of recession, many British High Streets have been described as declining into unprofitability, the bankruptcy of many national retail chains compounding the longer-term impacts of out-of-town retailing and the rise of lifestyle shopping. These 'failing' High Streets have become known through a negative language of dereliction and despair, indelibly associated with discount and 'distress' (read: working class) purchases. But in the rhetoric of those fighting to regenerate these High Streets—Mary Portas and the like—there's hope they can be revived by attracting a discerning middle-class clientele for whom malls seem to have limited appeal. This seemingly relies on the opening of art galleries, boutiques and coffee shops that will draw in those of a bohemian disposition, 'hipsters' looking for a consumer experience that's more interesting and 'authentic' than that offered in the contrived space of the mall. In short, it's suggested they can be remade, their cultural associations with distasteful, flawed consumption reworked by the replacement of discount stores with more upmarket ones that will ultimately produce a more resilient and successful High Street.

But the challenges here often seem immense. The levels of a vacancy on some High Streets are such that few appear prepared to take the risk of setting up new businesses without significant inducement or tax break

© The Editor(s) (if applicable) and The Author(s) 2017 **67**
P. Hubbard, *The Battle for the High Street*,
DOI 10.1057/978-1-137-52153-8_4

from local government, and in many cases, it has required a serious leap of faith to imagine that some local shopping streets can ever be revived. Recognizing this, Mary Portas (2011: 13) has argued 'High Streets must be ready to experiment, try new things, take risks and become destinations again…to be spaces and places that people want to be in'. Regenerating High Streets appears to rely on more than simply finding new occupants, requiring the reversal of long-standing images of decline and the construction of an atmosphere conducive to the attraction of a more affluent consumer base that will sustain new local shopping facilities. And it's this that raises the very real danger of gentrification, with policies intended to promote lively, vibrant and vital High Streets ultimately playing into the hands of those entrepreneurs and corporations for whom a declined High Street represents a prime development opportunity. This is something Heather McLean and colleagues have noted in the regeneration of Toronto's inner suburban shopping streets:

> Redevelopment proponents express a common desire to reinvent suburban commercial strips into "higher" value, "green" and "creative" neighbourhoods that emulate gentrified downtown commercial areas. They hope that regeneration initiatives will attract artists and middle class consumers of culture by combining infrastructure development with neighbourhood-scale efforts to reinvent streets with high-end coffee shops, bicycle repair facilities and farmers' markets. However, such strategies territorialize disinvented neighbourhoods, presenting them as empty and blighted, marking stores frequented by low-income residents as lacking and in need of improvement. In turn, these planning trends displace concerns about structural inequalities. (McLean et al. 2015: 1302–1303)

The suggestion here is that when stakeholders promote retail regeneration they are tacitly supporting gentrification and a revaluation of space that ultimately works in the interests of capital, not people. This is not an isolated phenomenon: one of the great contradictions of capitalism, as David Harvey (2011) has repeatedly pointed out, is that it has to devalue much of the fixed capital in a location before it can rebuild this landscape in a new, more profitable, form. Such is the logic of uneven development and the processes that encourage accumulation through dispossession. But in some towns and cities, this threat of dispossession seems so distant that the costs and benefits of regeneration for different groups are scarcely considered. Margate's High Street—routinely described as Britain's most derelict—is a case in point, a shopping street whose widespread description as blighted and broken preceded a sustained campaign of retail regeneration that now threatens to displace those whom it initially set out to assist.

Britain's Worst High Street

Summer 2014. I am in Margate, a sunny, Sunday morning, just before ten o'clock. I walk up and down the street, killing time before I am due to meet with a friend to take a walk along the coast. Occasionally, a car pulls over, someone gets out, wanders to the cashpoint, withdraws some money and then drives off. Slumped on a bench, a young man wearing sports casual gear shouts into a phone, asking where his friend disappeared to last night, and trying to secure a lift home, seemingly to no avail. *McDonalds* is open, but there's only one couple in there at this time of the morning. Nothing else appears open, so I am reduced to window-shopping, except, it seems, that not many windows have anything on display at all. Some are whitewashed and others are boarded up: *Paynes* the grocer, still proclaiming its status as Kent's largest independent fruitiers; a shop that used to sell 'cut priced' *Sweets & Mags*; *Shoe Express*, whose faded posters advertising closing-down sales have slipped down the window, crumpling at ground level; the more neatly shuttered *Woolworths*, next to the former *Clarks* shoe shop whose name is now obscured by a huge To Let sign. Rolling back the years, I find myself lapsing into the *modus operandi* of the A-level Geography student, marking off retail land use on a sketch map. All in all I count 28 abandoned and empty shops, around a third of all the retail premises in and around the High Street.

It's this prevalence of vacant shops that's caught the eye of the many journalists who have beat a path to town since its identification in 2009 as Britain's least successful High Street. In their rhetoric, the High Street mirrors the fortunes of the entire resort, a seaside town that is a shadow of its former self:

> In times gone by, a hot summer's day in the school holidays would have had retailers on Margate's High Street rubbing their hands with glee at the prospect of a steady flow of shoppers making a trip to the town centre, just a short walk from the seaside resort's sandy beach. But the benign conditions bring few shoppers to the town centre now. A stroll down the main strip quickly reveals why. Clusters of empty shop façades outnumber the surviving businesses in places. Faint lettering has left a reminder that the likes of *River Island* and *Marks & Spencer* have moved out. A *Woolworths* remains unoccupied. An array of charity shops and pound stores has filled some of the vacated units, the only outlets seemingly able to attract the dwindling numbers of customers. … Even its staunchest defenders have to concede that Margate is suffering from an acute case of High Street decline. (Savage 2009: 9)

These abandoned shops can be described in terms of ruination. They are 'sites which have not been exorcised, where the supposedly over-and-done with remains … they seethe with memories [*and*] haunt the visitor with vague intimations of the past, refusing fixity, and they also haunt the desire to pin memory down in place' (Edensor 2005: 829). And while many urban explorers and aesthetes portray abandoned urban sites as full of possibilities, vacant shops are more routinely described through negative metaphors of redundancy or waste. For, unlike other some other abandoned spaces in the contemporary city, vacant shops remain hermetically sealed, being haphazardly surveyed by security companies dedicated to frustrating any attempt at place-hacking or unsanctioned 'DIY urbanism' (Iveson 2013). They are not sites that can be appropriated by nature; they do not provide temporary accommodation for the homeless; no children play in them. Instead, their whitewashed windows and fading signs bear witness to changing economic circumstances, and the vicissitudes of contemporary capitalism that have rendered these premises functionally obsolete. Far from achieving the qualities of the sublime associated with classical ruins, these 'new ruins' are then understood only through discourses of dereliction (Bennett and Dickinson 2015).

In this sense, these empty shops—these unproductive *voids*—do not encourage the viewer to speculate on alternative urban futures, but rather evoke memories of the (all-too-recent) past. Clearly such memories are contingent given absent presences can produce varied emotions and suppositions depending on one's positionality (Holloway and Kneale 2008), but in the context of contemporary consumer landscapes, where retail trends and fashions are reflected in rapidly changing, fashionable store design and advertising, they are uncanny and disturbing sites. The boarded-up shop can summon forth memories—which cannot necessarily be easily articulated—of mundane and familiar acts of shopping and socializing, and juxtapose these with a present, in which such rituals appear to have been destroyed and lost, perhaps forever. As Tim Edensor (2005: 3) puts it, they are haunted precisely because 'the sudden force of the remembered but inexplicable impression or atmosphere rockets the past into the present, or conjures up an unidentifiable or even imaginary past'. The presence of ghostly remnants of an unfathomable past disturbs: a finger trace in the whitewashed windows proclaiming the 'last day' of opening, a faded poster for a circus that last visited months ago, the pile of yellowing circulars mounting on a door mat: all can stimulate a sense of loss for an imagined and idealized past (Fig. 4.1).

This is to argue that vacant shop units are more than just a statistical indicator of High Street vitalty and viability: they produce profound imaginings of loss and abandonment. In the case of Margate, each and every empty, abandoned or relict shop invokes the crowds and vitality of a (recent) time when it was a more thriving resort town, and bucket-and-spade tourism provided the town its *raison d'etre*. It triggers some dim and distant memories of a trip I made to the town in the 1970s with my parents, when we walked past the whelk stalls on the Sea front on our way to the High Street on a blisteringly hot day. I recall the High Street, not as one typified by 'butchers, bakers and candlestick makers', but a High Street where comparison and convenience shopping sat cheek-by-jowl with cultural, leisure and non-retail activities. A High Street that boasted *Burtons* for the gents (with a snooker hall above it, inevitably); *Dorothy Perkins* for women; *British Home Stores*, with a restaurant with a sea view; Bookshops, toy shops and record shops (*Our Price*); electrical stores (*Radio Rentals*) and a kitchenware shop; *Boots* the chemist; *WHSmiths* newsagents; *Woolworths*, with its pick and mix for the kids, cut-priced school clothes and the photo-booth where teens would gather to make 'selfies' long before the term had ever been coined; The *Wimpy* hamburger joint (fluorescent milkshakes and knickerbocker glory!); a

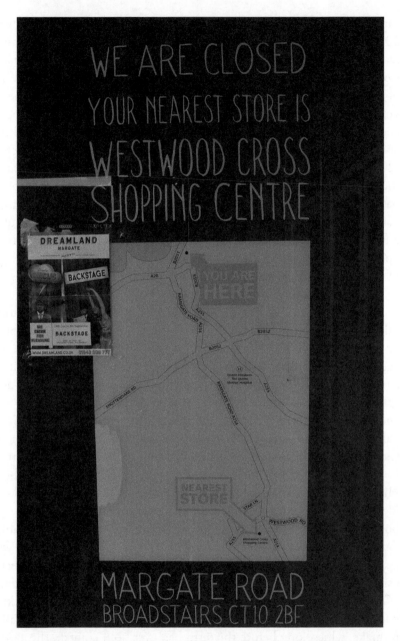

Fig. 4.1   Window display, former Primark store, Margate, 2015 (photo: author)

smattering of second-hand stores, perhaps, an antiques shop and a furniture store; A dry cleaners; Some hairdressers; One or two pubs, and several cafés; A High Street where there was something for everyone, where people of different classes and backgrounds could find something to suit their pocket; a vibrant and vital place.

The fact that the anticipated rapid redevelopment of the High Street (via processes of 'creative destruction') has not effaced these memories and hauntings of the recent past suggests the residents of Margate are, like me, being continually confronted by the past, and experiencing a sense of abandonment, of being out of time. This story of abandonment makes for good copy, and the British media has often taken a salacious delight in documenting the failure of Margate (and other High Streets like it), presenting the number of empty shops on the High Street as *prime facie* evidence of decline. This is narrated as a human as much as an economic tragedy. For what is evident from the photographs which the media use to inform us of Margate High Street's slow death is that the High Street remains populated: an unaccompanied mother pushes her pram determinedly; an old man pauses for breath on a bench, walking stick in hand; a man stares definitely at the camera grasping his shopping tightly, perhaps wondering why the photographer is so interested in the abandoned 'Cellular Phone' repair store. Such figures are indeterminate, but arguably, these are disadvantaged consumers, not the affluent, seduced white family consumers targeted by modern malls. Moreover, they are not the respectable working class of yesteryear, thrifty, community-oriented and worthy, who we might imagine thronging Margate High Street as tourists and residents in years gone by. Rather they appear to evoke a fragmented, imagined underclass of asylum seekers, the unemployed, single parents, the homeless and the vulnerable; an abandoned people, no less. No wonder, the press concluded, this was the area targeted by Nigel Farage and his English nationalist party UKIP in the 2015 General Election (Farage may have failed to gain the seat of Thanet South, but his party took the majority of seats on the local town council).

So, while approximately two-thirds of outlets in Margate remain open, the narration of the High Street as abandoned and ghostly is one in which characteristics of people and place are metaphorically and materially connected, presenting an unanswerable case for regeneration. The imagery and language are essentially one of abjection: Margate and its populations live in a world that appears both horrifying and pitiful to mainstream cultural commentators and media alike. The High Street is dying, and we are told that all that's left are businesses catering for an underclass. Here, narratives of neglect appear to evoke disgust through precisely the same processes that reproduce class divides, metaphors of waste being used to stigmatize working-class communities that, in turn, are incorporated into wider myths of 'no-go' Britain.

Streets of Disgust?

Margate represents a particularly interesting and much-cited example of High Street decline (and attempted regeneration) given this context of memory and loss. It's also one that gains resonance from the fact that the town is one of the most deprived areas in the generally affluent South East of England. This is reflected in the Office of National Statistics' Index of Multiple Deprivation, 2010 which places the town within the most deprived 20% of areas in England and Wales, with several wards close to the centre of Margate within the 5% of most deprived: Cliftonville West and Margate Central are among the top five most deprived neighbourhoods in Kent. Conventionally, this relative deprivation has been explained with reference to a number of factors, including the town's historic dependency on a declining tourism sector; a profoundly unbalanced housing market with high and increasing numbers of private rented properties; 'benefit-dependent' households in multiple occupation (Smith 2012); concentrations of children in care and other vulnerable groups; and high rates of both seasonal and long-term unemployment. There's also sometimes mention made of immigrant populations, and particularly those Eastern Europeans living in run-down ex-bed and breakfast accommodation. Here, it's notable that otherwise balanced official accounts of the fortunes of Margate have brought into a language of dereliction and despondency, the British Urban Regeneration Association speaking of the town as one of South East England's 'dumping grounds for people facing problems such as unemployment, social exclusion and substance abuse' (cited in Rickey and Houghton 2009: 47) and the Centre for Social Justice (2013: 12) describing it 'as struggling to stay above water since the 1960s when its tourist base dried up', being 'littered' with 'old hotels and guesthouses unsuitable for families'. At the extreme, the press has labelled Margate a 'recession-ravaged' and 'broken' town (*The Sun* 2010).

Margate, like several other notable British examples of retail decline, has become a metaphor regularly deployed in many journalistic depictions of the decline and fragmentation of working-class communities. In this coverage, there's frequent use of a language of defilement, with the dirt and decay of the High Street symbolizing the flawed values of local residents. Exploring how this language of disgust bleeds into the discourse of retail regeneration is particularly important given the working classes in Britain have long been victims of a symbolic violence that reduces their interests and lifestyles to a cliché. No longer 'respectable', the working class are known through a language which derides them as part of a 'feral underclass'—lazy, tacky and uncivilized, prone to violence and profoundly anti-social. It is a population widely depicted as prone to drunkenness, problem gambling and sexual immorality. Owen Jones (2012) concludes that the symbols and spaces of the working class have been reduced to a stereotype through the relentless derision of the behaviours and tastes of what is seen as a worthless, feckless group. Such discourses encourage everyone to aspire to, and identify with, middle-class values, driving a wedge between the haves and have-nots that is, perversely, no longer talked of in terms of class. In neoliberal societies, the great myth is that we can all be middle-class consumers so long as we are prepared to work hard. Morality and responsibility are hence emphasized over questions of access or discrimination in discussions of inequality.

Owen Jones' discussion of class and morality resonates with many other sociological readings of class transition, with the figure of the 'chav' having attracted considerable comment in recent times (e.g. Hayward and Yar 2006; Nayak 2006; Le Grand 2015). Suggesting that descriptions of the chav represent a contemporary inflection of a long-standing 'undeserving poor' discourse, a key theme in this work is that the language used to describe certain groups as socially marginalized, relies on metaphors of disgust, pollution and contamination. For example, Imogen Tyler (2013: 7) notes that established ways of speaking of the lower classes have been reanimated via 'a rush of descriptions of sullen, hooded, loitering, unemployed, pram-pushing, intoxicated youths', descriptions that reveal class disgust, contempt, and anxiety by dwelling on issues of embodiment and 'flawed' appearance. Elsewhere, connections are made between place and poverty to reinforce these myths. For example, in the controversial Channel Four documentary series *Benefits Street*, less affluent neighbourhoods are represented as insalubrious, dirty, overrun by litter, rats and dog-shit: their environmental character is mapped onto, and out of, the lives of those who live there. Such 'poverty porn' is, Tyler argues, not simply reactive but constitutive of social class because it fuels feelings of disgust among those who regard themselves as 'normal' (see also Jensen 2014).

Disgust, as Tyler (2013: 21) describes it, is an 'urgent, guttural and aversive emotion' which works, alongside other emotions, to create social distinctions of hierarchy and taste. This invocation of the notion of social abjection betrays Tyler's desire to distance the notion of disgust from a narrow understanding of disgust as an atavistic and primal reaction to that which literally endangers us. Instead, Tyler focuses on the feelings of disgust that we project upon those we are repeatedly told are a danger to society. This echoes the arguments of Martha Nussbaum (2004: 15), who seeks to distinguish between 'primary objects of disgust' ('the reminders of human animality and mortality: faeces, other bodily fluids, corpses, and animals') and the manipulation of this disgust by a dominant group that is seeking to cordon itself off from its own animality. Like Nussbaum, Tyler argues that, while disgust may retain some useful function in terms of avoiding danger, the linking of primary objects of disgust to particular social groups or populations is nearly always unhelpful. This moral disgust is, she argues, 'normatively irrational' as it does not help us identify what—or whom—is truly dangerous. Nonetheless, as geographer David Sibley (1995) has shown, it can be powerful in triggering defensive acts designed to shore up the boundaries between Self and Other, with the perceived violation of self-identity often manifested in exclusionary actions and strategies intended to 'cleanse' both society and space (see also Hubbard 2005b).

This move is significant in at least two senses. Firstly, it allows Tyler to hold to the power of disgust as a primal and visceral emotion that is intensely felt, and which circles around fears of contamination, pollution and despoilment. This positions abjection as a process that is inevitably about the policing of boundaries and struggles concerning the making of clear distinctions between Self and Other. Secondly, it allows Tyler to think about abjection as a socially lived process, which makes particular subjects the object of 'violent, objectifying disgust'. In simple terms, Tyler (2012: 5) is concerned with mapping 'the processes through which minoritised populations are imagined and configured as revolting and become subject to control, stigma and censure, and the practices through which individuals and groups resist, reconfigure and revolt against their abject subjectification'. In making such arguments, Tyler enriches the theoretical materials available for thinking about how the projection of negative values onto Others produces class division, extending analyses of class relations in contemporary Britain (e.g. Skeggs 1997; Haylett 2001; Lawler 2005; Nayak 2006) by revealing a continuing devaluation of working-class cultures created through repeated disgust reactions.

Here, it's worth noting that, the case for revivifying High Streets mirrors the more general argument put forward for urban redevelopment in which dirt and decay are associated with particular residents (and communities). As Ben Campkin's (2013) work on histories of urban renewal in London shows us, spaces are typically defined as in need of renewal and re-invention at times when their population is said to be the residuum of a once respectable (and 'clean') working-class population. The disgust expressed towards such populations justifies a remaking of place in which 'dirt' is swept away in a cleansing process that is, inevitably, also conceived as a civilizing process. As we have seen, retail regeneration policy contains similar moralizing tendencies, with deprivation per se obscured as a source of retail decline in discourses that, instead, place the blame for the decline of local shopping streets squarely on a residualized working class incapable of maintaining a High Street in the same way their predecessors did. Given that shopping practices are always informed by memories, and a nostalgic desire to recapture earlier times and places recalled as more orderly, cleaner and more sociable, this stigmatization of the current users of the High Street is understandable (Watson and Wells 2005). In this sense, it's hard to disagree with Tim Edensor's (2008: 331) assessment that 'the absent presence of an identifiable working class haunts romantic visions of the past but also those of future political programmes and assessments of the present, which complacently deny the continuing existence of a far more marginalized class'. Bluntly put, the current shoppers on High Streets like Margate's simply do not count, as it's these consumers who are perceived to have reduced it to a dirty, discount-dominated and declining shadow of its previous self.

Margate: Whose High Street?

Given that it has been regularly served up as one of Britain's worst High Streets, it was not surprising that Mary Portas visited Margate when 'fact finding': the poverty evident in the town, coupled with a 'failing' High Street appeared to support her model of a downwards spiral of decline in which local deprivation and weaker store performance combine to increase store closures. Equally unsurprising was the subsequent award of Portas Pilot status, and £100,000, to the town, one of twelve in the first tranche of funding in 2012. From the point of an award, this proved somewhat controversial. The filming of an episode of Channel Four's 'Save the High Street' in the town in 2012 was particularly contentious, with some members of the 'Town Team' resigning following rows about the ways the production team wanted to vet contributions to the programme, as well as concerns that the programme misrepresented the causes of retail decline (failing to mention the influence of the Westwood Cross shopping centre just ten minutes' drive away). Additionally, some residents and business representatives reacted badly to the involvement of locally born artist Tracey Emin in the documentary, and her suggestion Margate needed to capitalize on its existing slightly seedy reputation by marketing itself through the slogan, 'For a dirty weekend come to Margate'. Subsequently, in December 2012 *The Sunday Times*, under a Freedom of Information Act request, found that just £111.47 of the £100,000 allocated to the town had been spent on Margate's retailers in the first year of the pilot, while in June 2013 Portas herself criticized the decision by Eric Pickles, Minister of Communities and Local Government, to grant planning permission for a Tesco superstore on the seafront of Margate, an action she saw as undermining ambitions for regeneration, and indicative of the government's 'tepid' response to her report.

While the Portas initiative itself proved divisive, it clearly signaled an intention to regenerate Margate's High Street, with the Town Team's initial bid document spelling out a strategy based on creating a vibrant and attractive High Street built around food and arts, the cultivation of local heritage, and partnership working. Initial meetings of the Town Team in the former *Woolworths* building provided a forum in which initiatives designed to serve these ends were discussed, with pop-up shops, job clubs and 'have-a-go markets' mooted as ways of addressing some of these aims. In June 2013, the Margate Town Team Board decided to allocate £10,000 of the Mary Portas Funds to independent traders on the High Street who wanted to improve the look of their shop fronts; they also funded a 'singing windows' arts installation which piped birdsong onto the High Street from a number of store fronts, spent money on planting and cleaning and, in 2014, commissioned a new 'way-finding' project in collaboration with Thanet District Council and the Arts Council. *Southeastern* trains' donation of 500 free return tickets from London to Margate, and subsequent special £10 tickets, also provided a means to encourage visitors to come to the town and, hopefully, spend money on the High Street.

These initiatives, but more importantly perhaps, the opening of the Turner Gallery in 2011 (see Chap. 10), have succeeded in attracting new businesses to the town. Some have been extensively flagged in national media, such as *Roost*, an eatery offering locally sourced corn-fed chicken accompanied by rocket salad and homemade elderflower cordial, seemingly a world away from the vilified and ethnicized chicken shops that many local authorities are seeking to restrict from opening near schools because of fears about obesity and poor health (see Chap. 9). This restaurant was featured in men's style magazine *GQ's* 2015 'city guide' to Margate, which also highlighted *Breuer & Dawson* vintage shop; the conversion of the former *Superdrug* chemist into *The Sands* boutique hotel (established by an LSE graduate); and *Haeckels*, a business which makes cosmetics and beard oil products out of local seaweeds. In another (online) magazine *Civilian* ('Global Intelligence, Style and Culture') one reviewer offered over the top praise for the latter, arguing 'Dom Bridges— filmmaker, director and perfumer—is a perfect example of why Margate feels so exciting now. It's as if all of the reasons that I love this town beside the sea have been distilled, combined, balanced and enhanced.

Bridges and his global expansion-ready brand *Haeckels* are a working experiment perfectly reflecting the exciting direction that Margate is taking. In the grip of regeneration, the town and its inhabitants—whether the newly-arrived or those who have been here for generations—are on the cusp of … something' (Richards 2015: np) (Fig. 4.2).

Such hyperbole can meet with mixed reaction given the locals have long been used to their town being described as derelict, not a must-visit shopping destination for the hipster generation. For example, one new gourmet pizza restaurant ('*GB Pizza*') located close to the High Street has featured prominently in the media as evidence of the positive change instigated by the influx of 'new money', even featuring in some national newspaper articles highlighting the putative regeneration of the town. In one (now removed article) the owner spoke of herself as bringing to Margate the type of operation found in the trendier parts of London.

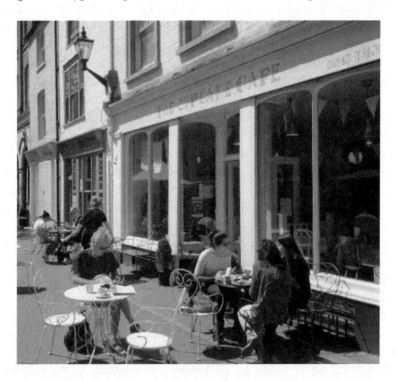

Fig. 4.2 Gentrified consumption, Margate Old Town (photo: author)

However, when she publicly spoke of overcoming 'Margate's issues'—such as 'grubby kids marauding the streets', 'lowlifes clutching tin of Tennent's Extra [*lager*]' and 'racist cab drivers and the in-your-face drug use'—there was something of a local backlash. For instance, one councilor went on record, to say he would boycott the restaurant, and others voiced similar displeasure:

> As has already been stated there's much truth in [*the owner's*] article but why did she have to adopt such a patronising tone—'… we're pretty sure visiting Londoners will spot the La Marzocco coffee machine and barrels from Borough Wines immediately'. I live in Thanet I know what a coffee machine and wine barrel looks like thanks very much. Think on … we're not all tattooed racists, some of us might have even been your customers! You need us as much as we need you. (Anonymous comment at http://birchington.blogspot.co.uk/2012/11/bbc-great-british-pizza-crisis.html, accessed May 2014)

These comments highlight the mutual resentments and distrusts evident across class lines, the residents of Margate characterized as addicted and dangerous, incoming Londoners as patronizing and effete. Irrespective, *GB Pizza* has been heralded as one of the signs that Margate is transforming from a drab seaside town into a bustling, hip art and food destination. The Town Team's Facebook page likewise highlights success stories: the opening of *Heidi's Crafts and Fabric* shop on the High Street following her initial trial in the collective Pop-up shop; *Morgan's Coffee Shop* with its lindyhop evenings; *Crafted Naturally* on Marine Drive; 'latte art' at the *Proper Coffee Shop* and so on. Many of these offer a range of ethnicized cuisines or fashions, and embody varied forms of cosmopolitanism, but they are overwhelmingly run by the white middle class, not ethnic entrepreneurs from Margate's immigrant population, which includes large numbers of recent Polish, Latvian and Romanian arrivals, as well as more established Caribbean, Pakistani and Bangladeshi groups (the number in the Black and Ethnic Minority population more than doubling in the decade 2001–2011 to reach 6000). Here, it's worth quoting from Sharon Zukin et al. (2009: 62), who conclude that high-end art galleries, vintage boutiques and cafés provide a material base for new kinds of cosmopolitanism 'that ignore old expressions of ethnic homogeneity and contrast with cultural forms, including consumption spaces, which embody low-status identities'. These forms are, in a very real sense, abject, with their effacement and replacement by white, middle-class aspirational 'hipster' stores unequivocally depicted as regeneration rather than the gentrification that it amounts to.

The suggestion from the US literature is that race and ethnicity are as important as class for understanding retail change, with a language of exclusion sometimes suggesting clear limits to whom is perceived to belong on particular shopping streets. In North American cities the long-standing division of black and white populations is particularly important, albeit some studies note a fracturing of the black population between those poorer residents who oppose gentrification and those middle-class blacks who might be part of the gentrification process itself (Moore 2009; Kasinitz and Zukin 2016). These North American studies point to the complex ways retail capital can be caught up in ethnic struggles over space and place, entwining with culture in somewhat unpredictable ways. Sarah Schulman's (2012) acid invocation of changes in New York's Alphabet City on the East Side is indicative:

> These new business ... would be open and one day then immediately packed, as though the yuppies were waiting in holding pens to be transported en masse to new, ugly expensive places. Quickly the battle was on and being waged block by block until the original tenants had almost nowhere left to go to pay the prices they could afford for food and the items they recognized and like. So the *Orchidia* [*an Italian/Ukrainian deli*] was replaced by a *Steve's Ice Cream*, then a *Starbucks* ... The corner bodega that sold tamarind, plantain and yucca was replaced by an upscale deli that sells Fuji water, the emblematic yuppie product. The Polish butcher was replaced by a suburban bar. Now if I want to buy fresh meat or fish, I have to go to Whole Foods (known as 'Whole Paycheck') which is ten blocks away. Rents in my building have gone from $205 a month to $2800 per month. And to add insult to injury, these very square new businesses that were culturally bland, parasitic and very American coded themselves as 'cool' or 'hip' when they were the opposite. (Schulman 2012: 33)

This devastating account of the cultural and ethnic change signaled by retail transformation has been confirmed by many others who suggest that white incomers to US inner city districts often describe established non-white and immigrant businesses as aesthetically displeasing, or chaotic. And while it's tempting to suggest that this is a peculiarly US phenomena, European examples of inner city retail change indicate similarly racist imaginations are often in play (see Everts and Jackson 2009; Hentschel and Blokland 2016).

The ethnicized dimensions of retail change in Margate are perhaps less sharply apparent, but the observation that many of the new stores taken to herald Margate's retail renaissance are run by white hipster incomers is an important one. Indeed, Mary Portas and others have repeatedly pointed to the Old Town of Margate as providing the model for retail regeneration, suggesting High Street can successfully mimic its blend of boho art galleries, coffee shops and vintage boutiques. There's never any mention of nearby Cliftonville, where Northdown Road offers a different vision of a thriving shopping street, with its Sri Lankan curry house, Caribbean food shop, Halal butchers, Polish grocery stores, estate agents offering cheap lets, scooter and bike shops, pharmacies and a post office. The idea that High Streets need to reflect multicultural Britain is important, but many potential models of 'cosmopolitan retailing' appear to be ignored in the dominant atmosphere of austerity nostalgia that privileges 1950s vintage furniture, pie and mash and 'proper' beer over the cultural imports of the more recent past.

The suggestion here is that contemporary middle-class notions of 'cosmopolitan' identity are highly circumscribed. This given, at a time when concepts of 'diversity' and 'mixed-use' High Streets are 'rendered in rather reductive-instrumentalist terms as being socially desirable' (Griffiths et al. 2008: 1177), it's important to question whether these very notions are themselves based on an essentially middle-class view of diversity and inclusion. Steven Miles (2012) concurs, arguing we need to be wary in terms of buying into myths of urban conviviality given that positive images of cosmopolitan shopping streets perpetuate a myth of shared prosperity, rather than what is likely to be the more uncomfortable reality that lies beneath. This is something that becomes obvious to me when I witness a black woman in her sixties wandering into the *Real Coffee* company in Margate and asking for a white coffee. The youngish bearded male barista asked her if she meant latte, flat white, or cappuccino? She looked a little befuddled, and repeated, 'Just a white coffee'.

He then asked which bean, offering Colombian or Peruvian? Again, the woman looked a bit puzzled, and plumped for the Peruvian. The coffee duly arrived, but when the women asked for sugar, the barista told her that she should not as the bean was naturally quite sweet. She appeared embarrassed, and quickly left the café clutching her (expensive) coffee.

Witnessing this type of transaction, it's easy to see how retail change can displace long-term users of local shopping streets. When these groups feel 'out of place', and shops no longer cater for their tastes, or budgets, then, as Peter Marcuse (1985) argues, the pressure on them to go elsewhere is considerable. This type of wholesale transition is yet to happen in Margate, but it's certainly threatening to happen. Indeed, it's already possible to witness cultural conflicts occurring which are akin to those described in the wider literature on retail gentrification. Yet it's understandably hard for those who have opened the new cafés and boutiques that have popped up along the High Street, to regard their own presence in the town as in any way negative. As Phil Kazinitz and Sharon Zukin (2016) argue, those opening new stores in inner city neighbourhoods do not just see themselves as economic entrepreneurs, but cultural entrepreneurs, keen to date the transformation of these areas to their own arrival, proclaiming a moral ownership of the street in the process. In the streets of New York they discuss, it's gentrifiers who have made the street safer 'for all', despite the fact their presence has effaced much of the class and ethnic diversity that existed previously. The changing 'character' of a local shopping street is hence shaped by such claims to space, and the use of a language which contrasts the green, healthy nature of new businesses with the dirty or disordered nature of the ones they replaced. Notions of value and distinction are always in play, with classed dispositions hidden under the surface of these categories (Bourdieu 1984).

The nascent gentrification of Margate's High Street, and lack of resistance that's been expressed to this, is then cause for concern. Experiences in the USA and elsewhere suggest we need to remain wary of the boutiquing of High Streets, and attempts to revive them by providing facilities which might be more valued by middle-class consumers than existing residents, particularly immigrants and less affluent populations. While Margate's High Street has routinely been described as 'dead' or 'dying', it still remained important in the lives of many local residents, who used it as a space for meeting-up and socializing, hunting for bargains in charity shops, taking a break in the perennially busy *Costa Coffee*, or picking up a prescription from the chemists. This is to make a crucial point: High Streets are not just about shopping, but are also social spaces. In this sense, while the rise of vacant properties on Margate's High Street was a clear cause for concern, whether the occupation of these premises by pop-up art galleries or vintage stores has improved the High Street more than the addition of a fast food takeaway, a tattoo parlour, a betting shop, or a chain pubs is a matter for debate. In terms of 'sociality', as well as economic viability, we need to critically question what new stores add to local shopping streets serving the less affluent. Here, it's important to stress that, even before the 'retail revolution' of the 1980s and 1990s, shopping was never the majority activity on the High Street. This suggests a need to think about the interdependence between retail and community services, housing, offices and commerce that can create a sustainable mixed use High Street (Jones et al. 2007), as well as recognizing the importance of 'third spaces'—those unassuming semi-public spaces between home and work where people can meet and socialize—that are particularly important in deprived areas (Hickman 2013; Warner et al. 2013).

I will return to Margate later in the book in the light of these arguments, questioning whether its nascent regeneration via the emergence of hipster businesses provides any sort of model of sustainable retail revival. But in the immediately following chapters, my intention is not so much to focus on the consequences of retail change, but to explore the notions of community and identity invoked via visions of the desirable and inclusive High Street that have been worked through in other British contexts. As in Margate, concerns about vacant and derelict shops are often to the fore, but in many cases locally specific discourses have focused instead on the premises thought 'out of place' on contemporary High Streets, with these depicted as objects of disgust standing in the way of regeneration. In each case, this disgust appears to be related to the perceived transgression of gentrified, middle-class norms of behaviour and comportment, with those who frequent betting shops, fast food takeaways, lap dance clubs, tanning shops, nail bars or bargain booze off licences regarded as exhibiting flawed, unhealthy forms of consumption. In each case, both good taste and morality are considered to have been violated, with the consequence of this being a specific linking of the personal and the social: those feeling disgusted are constituted as respectable—albeit 'anxious and defensive'—middle-class subjects (Lawler 2005: 443). It's this which makes it so hard to criticize the regeneration of the High Street: if we do not acquiesce to dominant visions of the 'good' High Street, we risk being shown up as lacking class, distinction and taste.

References

Bennett, L. and Dickinson, J. (2015). Forcing the empties back to work? Ruinphobia and the bluntness of law and policy. Paper at Transience and Permanence in Urban Development workshop, January 2015 at the University of Sheffield.

Bourdieu, P. (1984). *Distinction: A social critique of the judgment of taste.* Cambridge: Harvard University Press.

Campkin, B. (2013). *Remaking London: Decline and regeneration in urban culture.* London: IB Tauris.

Centre for Social Justice (2013). *Turning the tide: Social justice in five seaside towns.* London: Centre for Social Justice.

Edensor, T. (2005). The ghosts of industrial ruins: Ordering and disordering memory in excessive space. *Environment and Planning D: Society and Space, 23*(6), 829–849.

Edensor, T. (2008). Mundane hauntings: Commuting through the phantasmagoric working-class spaces of Manchester, England. *Cultural Geographies, 15*(3), 313–333.

Everts, J., & Jackson, P. (2009). Modernisation and the practices of contemporary food shopping. *Environment and Planning D: Society and Space, 27*(5), 917–935.

Griffiths, S., Vaughan, L., Haklay, M. M., & Jones, E. C. (2008). The sustainable suburban High Street: A review of themes and approaches. *Geography Compass, 2*(4), 1155–1188.

Harvey, D. (2011). *The enigma of capital and the crisis of capitalism.* London: Profile Books.

Haylett, C. (2001). Illegitimate subjects? Abject whites, neoliberal modernisation and middle class multiculturalism. *Environment and Planning D: Society and Space., 19*(3), 351–370.

Hayward, K., & Yar, M. (2006). The 'chav' phenomenon: Consumption, media and the construction of a new underclass. *Crime, Media, Culture, 2*(1), 9–28.

Hentschel, C., & Blokland, T. (2016). Life and death of the great regeneration vision: Diversity, decay, and upgrading in Berlin's ordinary shopping streets. In S. Zukin, P. Kasinitz, & X. Chen (Eds.), *Global cities, local streets*. New York: Routledge.

Hickman, P. (2013). "Third places" and social interaction in deprived neighbourhoods in Great Britain. *Journal of Housing and the Built Environment*, *28*(2), 221–236.

Holloway, J., & Kneale, J. (2008). Locating haunting: A ghost-hunter's guide. *Cultural Geographies*, *15*(3), 297–312.

Hubbard, P. (2005b). 'Inappropriate and incongruous': Opposition to asylum centres in the English countryside. *Journal of Rural Studies*, *21*(1), 3–17.

Iveson, K. (2013). Cities within the city: Do-it-yourself urbanism and the right to the city. *International Journal of Urban and Regional Research*, *37*(3), 941–956.

Jensen, T. (2014). Welfare commonsense, poverty porn and doxosophy. *Sociological Research Online*, 19(3), http://www.socresonline.org.uk/19/3/3.html

Jones, O. (2012). *Chavs: The demonization of the working class*. London: Verso.

Jones, P., Roberts, M., & Morris, L. (2007). *Rediscovering mixed-use streets: The contribution of local High Streets to sustainable communities*. Bristol: Policy Press/Joseph Rowntree Foundation.

Kasinitz, P., & Zukin, S. (2016). From ghetto to global: Two neighbourhood shopping streets in New York City. In S. Zukin, P. Kasinitz, & X. Chen (Eds.), *Global cities, local streets*. New York: Routledge.

Lawler, S. (2005). Class, culture and identity. *Sociology*, *39*(5), 797–806.

Le Grand, E. (2015) Linking moralization and class: The role of ressentiment and respectability in the social reaction to chavs. Sociological Research Online, 20(4), 15, http://www.socresonline.org.uk/20/4/15.html

Marcuse, P. (1985). Gentrification, abandonment and displacement: Connections, causes and policy responses in New York City. *Journal of Urban and Contemporary Law*, *28*(1), 195–240.

McLean, H., Rankin, K., & Kamizaki, K. (2015). Inner-suburban neighbourhoods, activist research, and the social space of the commercial street. *ACME: An International E-Journal for Critical Geographies*, *14*(4), 1283–1308.

Miles, S. (2012). The neoliberal city and the pro-active complicity of the citizen consumer. *Journal of Consumer Culture*, *12*(2), 216–230.

Moore, K. S. (2009). Gentrification in black face? The return of the black middle class to urban neighborhoods. *Urban Geography*, *30*(2), 118–142.

Nayak, A. (2006). Displaced masculinities: Chavs, youth and class in the post-industrial city. *Sociology, 40*(5), 813–831.

Nussbaum, M. (2004). *Hiding from Humanity: Shame, disgust, and the law.* Princeton: Princeton University Press.

Portas, M. (2011). The Portas review: An independent review into the future of our High Streets. http://www.maryportas.com/news/2011/12/12/the-portas-review/

Richards, L. (2015) Made of Margate. 14 January. http://civilianglobal.com/features/made-of-margate-haeckels-best-beard-oil-dom-bridges/

Rickey, B., & Houghton, J. (2009). Solving the riddle of the sands: Regenerating England's seaside towns. *Journal of Urban Regeneration & Renewal, 3*(1), 46–55.

Savage, M. (2009). How the recession turned Margate into a ghost town. *The Independent* 15 August, p. 9.

Schulman, S. (2012). *The gentrification of the mind: Witness to a lost imagination.* Berkeley: University of California Press.

Sibley, D. (1995). *Geographies of exclusion: Society and difference in the west.* London: Routledge.

Skeggs, B. (1997). *Formations of class & gender: Becoming respectable.* London: Sage.

Smith, D. P. (2012). The social and economic consequences of housing in multiple occupation (HMO) in UK coastal towns: Geographies of segregation. *Transactions of the Institute of British Geographers, 37*(3), 461–476.

The Sun (2010). How tide has turned on Margate, 20 March, http://www.the-sun.co.uk/sol/homepage/features/2850536/How-Margate-has-fallen-from-popular-resort-to-broken-town.html

Tyler, I. (2013). The riots of the underclass? Stigmatisation, mediation and the government of poverty and disadvantage in neoliberal Britain. *Sociological Research Online, 18*(4), 6.

Tyler, M. (2012). 'Glamour girls, macho men and everything in between': Un/doing gender and dirty work in Soho's sex shops. In R. Simpson, N. Slutskaya, P. Lewis, & H. Höpfl (Eds.), *Dirty work: Concepts and identities.* Basingstoke: Palgrave Macmillan.

Warner, J., Talbot, D., & Bennison, G. (2013). The café as affective community space: Reconceptualizing care and emotional labour in everyday life. *Critical Social Policy, 33*(2), 305–324.

Watson, S., & Wells, K. (2005). Spaces of nostalgia: The hollowing out of a London market. *Social & Cultural Geography, 6*(1), 17–30.

Zukin, S., Trujillo, V., Frase, P., Jackson, D., Recuber, T., & Walker, A. (2009). New retail capital and neighborhood change: Boutiques and gentrification in New York City. *City & Community, 8*(1), 47–64.

5

24-Hour Party People

Much of the rhetoric surrounding High Streets focuses on their importance as daytime spaces of shopping and sociality, with relatively little attention given to its use after dark. For all this, British High Streets have been profoundly shaped in the last couple of decades by the increasing vibrancy of their nighttime offer, with specific licensing reforms encouraging more pubs, clubs, and restaurants to open. As we will see, these venues have created jobs and added a certain liveliness to the High Street in the evening and at night, but they often exist in conflict with daytime uses, with the transition between the daytime and nighttime often witnessing significant changes in the feel and atmosphere of some local 'shopping streets'. One general tendency here is for the street to become more dominated by younger people as older ones retreat, and for any semblance of 'family' atmosphere to be overwhelmed by an edgier vibe that appears off-putting to those sensitized by media stories of alcohol-fuelled excess, violence and anti-sociality.

The nighttime economy, once heralded as the potential savior of failing High Streets, has hence been portrayed in many policy documents as a deadweight dragging down the reputation of particular town and city centres. Mary Portas' review of High Streets confirms as much, insisting

© The Editor(s) (if applicable) and The Author(s) 2017
P. Hubbard, *The Battle for the High Street*,
DOI 10.1057/978-1-137-52153-8_5

leisure uses might become more important in the future of High Streets, but offering few recommendations to better integrate nighttime and daytime activities. However, elsewhere there's been a more sustained discussion of how the High Street at night might fit into current visions of a more inclusive, leisured, High Street that is welcoming to all, both day and night. Local planning and licensing regulation has been integral here, encouraging the opening of venues favouring 'cosmopolitan' consumption—e.g. craft gin, US microbrews and gourmet burgers–over those offering a narrower diet of discount alcohol and cheap food. While the latter tend to be viewed as the haunt of 'flawed' consumers whose presence threatens the moral order of nightlife, the former are explicitly figured as associated with a privileged and discerning class habitus. Encouraging one over the other is a blatant example of social engineering on the High Street, an attempt to court the 'creative class' (Florida 2002) at the expense of the working class. In this chapter, I argue that this putative 'remoralization of the night' is an important, but little-noted dimension of urban gentrification, one with significant implications for High Streets in contemporary Britain.

Inventing the Nighttime Economy

The city at night has long been known (and even celebrated) for its capacity to offer conviviality, and its excessive liveliness is also something that can arouse fear. Socially, this has meant that many of the individuals, populations and 'figures' routinely encountered in the daytime city can take on new and even sinister meanings in the city at night. Indeed, social historians such as Lynda Nead (2000), Wolfgang Schivelbusch (1988), Joachim Schlör (1998) and Matthew Beaumont (2015) make the point that prior to the 'industrialization of light', any individual wandering the streets at night was treated with a certain suspicion, assumed to be dangerous or deviant in some way. Curfew was the preferred tool to deal with such characters and a means to distinguish between the respectable and those whose motives were more suspect. This cemented the association of night, criminality and immorality. For example, any woman who was on a dark street without an escort was regarded as a prostitute, a 'woman of the streets', while men walking alone were considered to be vagrant, if not an outright criminal.

The mass illumination of the city and the beginnings of industrialized 'night-life' in the nineteenth-century metropolis profoundly changed this, as William Sharpe notes:

> The installation of gaslight in London's West End in 1807 ignited a series of innovations that permanently rearranged the rhythms of everyday life, transforming traditional patterns of industry, commerce, leisure, and consumption. The concept of "nightlife" was born, along with the twenty-four-hour workday. With reliable lighting came safer streets, late shopping, and vastly expanded entertainments. The illumination of the city changed the very way people thought about—and thus lived in—the night. Darkness, so long a barrier to human activity, quickly became a stimulant. (Sharpe 2008: 17)

Eric Monkkonen (1981: 541) concurs, noting that nighttime in the late nineteenth- and early twentieth-century city was characterized by the relatively intense use of public space by 'people of all classes'. Pubs, cafés, restaurants, dance halls, theatres and music halls provided a variety of leisure opportunities which enlivened streets that were mainly used for shopping during the daytime, with cinemas later emerging as the most urban of all leisure forms, affordable to the working classes but also frequented by the more affluent (Zukin 1998). *Odeon* cinemas appeared on many British High Streets, their Modern art deco forms marking them out as stylish and of-the-moment. Such venues ensured town centres remained a fairly energetic and vibrant place at night, with nightlife being produced and consumed by the 'masses'.

However, in the 1980s and 1990s, the realization many were prepared to travel out of town for their consumption needs challenged the preeminence of town and city centres as sites of nighttime sociality. New peripheral and ex-urban sites of consumption began to appear. As we have seen, the emergence of 'Family Entertainment Complex'—a collection of restaurants anchored by a multiplex cinema and bowling alley—changed patterns in cinema-going in the UK in the 1990s, effectively marking the death-nail of the in-town 'cinema', a space that no longer appeared modern but was more routinely described, in disparaging terms, as a 'flea pit'. Like the retail mall, the multiplex was read as a quintessentially post-modern form, offering a variety of films catering for different audiences and taste cultures, effectively rejecting the pleasures of mass consumption. It was also understood as clean, safe, and comfortable, and easily accessible to the car-borne consumer, who no longer had to worry about town centre parking. In this sense, while the High Street cinemas that provided the focus for urban leisure in the 1930s through to the 1980s were a thoroughly urban phenomenon, the multiplex appeared 'ex-urban'. Rather than keeping audiences in touch with metropolitan ways of life, the multiplex turned its back on the city, creating a form of leisure that was distinctly placeless but immensely popular, especially with white, middle-class consumers (Hubbard 2003).

One of the first policy responses to this perceived flight of consumers 'out of town' was the attempted reinvention of town and city centres as 24-hour *playscapes* (Chatterton and Hollands 2003). Key to this idea was that ailing High Streets—particularly in the de-industrializing cities of the North and Midlands—could be revivified by focusing on their evening and nighttime economies, with the cities of continental Europe providing the inspiration (especially Barcelona, whose vibrant cultures of eating and drinking were especially highlighted at the time of the 1992 Olympics). But this focus on regenerating the High Street through an improved nightlife offer played to other agendas, most notably a 'creative city' thesis suggesting culture could be one of the key drivers of the post-industrial economy (a theme I return to in Chap. 10). Here, the burgeoning appetite both for weekend 'urban tourism' and the rise of corporatized 'dance' and DJ culture pointed to the potential contribution that nighttime businesses—notably clubs, pubs, hotels and cafés—might make to local economies. The fact that many of the jobs created might be poorly paid ones involving unsociable hours was rarely noted, even though there's plentiful academic evidence suggesting those working in the evening economy have poorer diets than those who work in the day, are pre-disposed to stress and are more likely to smoke and drink (Norman 2011).

Talk of the nighttime economy was hence to the fore in the Labour government's 1990s urban regeneration agenda, with its vision of an 'urban renaissance' based on 'romantic visions which looked forward to a time when British cities had shed their dour industrial pasts to be re-born as fully European: relaxed, cosmopolitan and urbane' (Hadfield 2006: 6). Partly in response to the rise of out of town malls and leisure parks, this was a vision in which struggling daytime High Streets were reimagined as bustling, vibrant entertainment zones in which a continental

European-style café culture would encourage residents and visitors alike to dwell long after the traditional 5 pm closing time when the majority of commercial activity ceased. This was a vision predicated on particular notions of democratic and shared space. As planning expert Marion Roberts (2004: 13) writes, even if the term urban renaissance was often loosely specified, it was widely taken to refer to 'a revitalisation of towns and cities in a traditionally European model, where urban areas and in particular, town and city centres became inclusive places where people live, work and participate in leisure activities on a harmonious basis'.

Market deregulation was the key means the government used to promote the nighttime economy, particularly the loosening of the licensing laws. The key legislation—the *Licensing Act 2003*—was lauded in many quarters for sweeping away much of the bureaucracy that discouraged licensed activities such as the sale of alcohol, the provision of late-night entertainment and serving of food on the High Street. In effect, this Act brought together the existing licensing regimes to create a single 'licensed premise' system in an effort to encourage new applications, while also allowing local authorities significantly more discretion in terms of setting permitted opening hours. The latter was in part an attempt to encourage a more relaxed ambience in British town and city centres where the traditional 11 pm closing time appeared to promote binge drinking at 'last orders', and often led to a rush for taxis and public transport at a time these services were not particularly well placed to cope.

In many ways, this deregulation worked, at least in terms of encouraging more consumers onto the High Street in the evening. At the same time rural pub numbers continued to tumble (Andrews and Turner 2012), the Institute of Alcohol Studies documented a steady rise in the number of on-premise alcohol licences in England and Wales from 2003 onwards, with a total of 204,000 by 2013. While the number of '24 hour' or post-11 pm licenses remain a relatively small proportion of these—roughly 10% of the total—there has also been a steady increase year-on-year, with most of these venues being in town and city centres. In short, there are now more licensed premises on the High Street, and more open for longer. These venues have created jobs and revenue and have become significant drivers of the local economy, especially in the provincial capitals (e.g. Newcastle, Leeds and Manchester) most renowned for their vibrant nightlife.

But far from producing the relaxed urbanity taken as the characteristic of continental European cities after dark, the nighttime economy today is depicted as dominated by a particular form of consumption: alcohol-centric, youth-oriented and relentlessly commercial. Criminologists Keith Hayward and Dick Hobbs (2007: 449) argue that the traditional bars that catered to a wide clientele have, by and large, been replaced by national chains which stripped their premises of 'unnecessary encumbrances such as tables and chairs', providing affordable but high-strength lagers and ciders, shots and 'buzz drinks' to a new generation of 'psychoactive consumers' in 'an invitation to transgress'. These 'vertical drinking' establishments 'deliberately and shrewdly' targeted young people, encouraging a 'reckless form' of hedonistic consumer culture that may be damaging both to themselves and to others (Hayward and Hobbs 2007: 450). Violence has certainly been depicted as endemic in and around this new generation of nightlife spaces: the 2001/02 British Crime Survey found 21% of all violent incidents in Britain occurred in or around a pub or club, and 38% of violence between strangers occurred in that location (Allen et al. 2005). The peak time for the attendance of patients with assault-related injuries was between nine on Friday evening and three on Saturday morning (Finney 2004).

Consequently, the significant measures taken to promote the nighttime economy of British cities have been the subject of a sustained media backlash, with attempts to create vibrant '24 hour cities' accused of rendering the High Street more mono-cultural by promoting a high-volume 'vertical' drinking culture associated with youthful excess and violence. Stories concerning the antics of Philip Laing, who drunkenly urinated on a war memorial following a student pub crawl in 2009, or the tale of Wendy Lewis—dubbed Britain's 'most disgusting woman' following her arrest for performing a drunken sex act on Blackpool's seafront cenotaph—were just the tip of the iceberg as the media whipped up a moral panic about the loutish behaviour of revelers in 'binge Britain' (see Campbell 2012; Hubbard 2013); all a far cry from the descriptions of cultured 24-hour cities to the fore in the urban scholarship of the 1990s (e.g. Landry and Bianchini 1995; Lovatt and O'Connor 1995).

So, while policies promoting nightlife were successful in the sense they made hedonistic, alcohol-fuelled nightlife cultures more popular and accessible than ever before, the flipside of this was increased late-night criminality and anti-sociality. No wonder the Department for Communities and Local Government (2012: 6) felt it fit to report in its response to Mary Portas' Review that 'our town centres often become no-go zones when shops close and pubs open, leading to the blight of anti-social behaviour that keeps people away and causing the High Street to go into a spiral of decline'. But 'no go' for whom? Clearly not for those who frequent clubs and pubs in town and city centres every weekend. But in Rosemary Bromley et al.'s (2000) study of safety concerns in the late-night city centre, the elderly expressed particular anxieties about 'drink-dominated' High Streets, with the proliferation of pubs and clubs on certain High Streets heightening fears among this population about using these. Elsewhere, the gendered dimensions of this anxiety have also been highlighted: women have been increasingly targeted by the nightlife industries (e.g. through drinks promotions, discounted entry fees and female-friendly policies such as women bouncers and free minibuses home), but nightlife is accused of being a repository of casual misogyny and sexism. The extent to which this encourages sexual assault remains a matter of considerable debate (e.g. see Burgess et al. 2009 and Brooks 2013, for different views of the 'moral panic' around drinks spiking) but the consequence is that many women simply avoid going out (Hubbard 2013). In Deborah Talbot's work (2011), the racialized nature of nightlife is also highlighted, with the enactment of the 2003 Licensing Act accused of closing down spaces for subcultural expression associated. As Talbot details, the licensing policies of most local authorities (and the associated 'juridification' of nightlife) favour corporate chains over the 'alternative' or even community-run venues associated with non-white populations. Here, the notorious 696 form required by the Metropolitan police in advance of any music event has been accused of marginalizing 'grime' music and other genres particularly associated with non-white groups, meaning these scenes have been spatially and socially excluded.

So, while the rise of the evening economy has seen large numbers return to the High Street at night, there's still considerable discussion about the exclusions this has set in motion (Hadfield 2006). Within these debates, issues concerning class have often been glossed over. Speaking of the anti-sociality associated with alcohol consumption, Keith Hayward and Dick Hobbs (2007: 452) argue that 'six pints of lager or a bottle of champagne can produce a transgressive pharmacological and cultural nexus that is not class-specific'. Consequently, they argue, 'binge drinking and its associated transgressions' are not explicitly linked to class, this type of behaviour being seen as the default for younger consumers irrespective of their socio-economic status. Perhaps there's some truth in this, as there's no clear evidence problematic drinking is isolated to any particular class faction in the UK today (Brierley-Jones et al. 2014). After all, wine consumption in the home—often cited as a source of distinction and the display of cultural capital by middle-class consumers (Holloway et al. 2008)—has been identified as a widespread form of damaging drinking. However, it's the harmful effects of 'Mass Volume Vertical Drinking' on our High Streets—as opposed to alcohol dependency in the home—that is emphasized by the media, with 'working class' venues and streets particularly disparaged. This points to the class dynamics, and hypocrisy, involved in the regulation of alcohol consumption, the vilification of city centre pubs offering cut-price drinks being a particular case in point. Arguments for minimum alcohol pricing, the imposition of saturation zones and tighter licensing laws are then regularly mooted as ways of 'disciplining' the working class into civilized middle-class forms of comportment (Roberts and Eldridge 2007; Haydock 2014).

Class and Alcohol in the Nighttime City

When comedians poke fun at the 'British disease' of binge drinking, *Wetherspoons* is normally the punchline. Whilst not the largest pub chain in the UK, it's perhaps the most recognizable given its 900-plus pubs share a strong brand identity, typically located on High Streets but much larger than the traditional High Street pub. Many are architecturally distinguished, being ex-bank buildings (e.g., *The Beckett's Bank* in Leeds or *The Bank House*, Cheltenham), cinemas (e.g., *The Peter Cushing* in Whitstable, located in the former Oxford cinema and bingo hall) or post offices (*The Last Post* in Southend-on-Sea). Behind their sometimes grand façades, the interiors are not snug, but open-plan, with large numbers of tables set up for eating and drinking throughout the day, arrayed around a capacious central drinking area and characteristically lengthy bar. *Wetherspoons* is noted for its early opening, boasting it's the only large pub firm that opens all its pubs early in the morning, serving 350,000 breakfasts and 750,000 hot drinks per week (some pubs open as early as seven in the morning). However, the chain is perhaps best known for its competitive pricing, serving 'real' ale and cask beers often at discount prices: there's usually a beer available for £1.99 (elsewhere on the High Street, this is typically in the region of £3 to £5): bottles of wine are typically on offer for less than ten pounds, and there are regular meal offers such as steak and chips with a drink for £8. Coffee can be as little as a pound with a chocolate biscuit thrown in for good measure. Combined with free wi-fi, and a lack of intrusive music, it's little wonder these premises attract a diverse audience: market traders and nightshift workers at breakfast, pensioners and shoppers popping in for mid-morning coffee, parents with young children in the afternoon, perhaps after the school run, and then, later in the evening, students and groups of younger adults who might be visiting as part of a pub crawl or who are on the way to a club, alongside the more hardened sessional drinkers who treat the pub as their 'local'.

It's, therefore, tempting to equate *Wetherspoons* in the twentieth century to the coffee houses of the eighteenth and nineteenth century that Jurgen Habermas (1991) and other commentators identified as the quintessential public sphere, a space that is open and affordable to all, regardless of rank and privilege. Although *Wetherspoons* have been praised for their inclusive ethos, support for locally sourced 'real ales', and bringing abandoned High Street premises back into use (Brearley 2014), their plans to open new pubs often face stiff local opposition. Most of this is classic NIMBY stuff: local residents, perhaps mindful of property prices, allege these pubs will create noise and nuisance that will reduce local amenity values. The fact that the pubs open beyond midnight at weekends, and create parking problems throughout the week, is regularly cited by those seeking to prevent their opening. But others draw particular attention to the problems of adding more alcohol provision to the High Street. For example, London Road Action Group in Brighton objected in May 2015 to the conversion of disused Co-Operative food store to a *Wetherspoons* pub on the basis they did not want to see London Road (a Portas Pilot High Street) become an 'alcohol-led economy' like Brighton's notorious West Street, which boasts a strip of pubs and nightclubs from the city's train station down to the seafront. In the event, planning permission was refused, with hundreds of objection letters (including one from local Green MP Caroline Lucas) stressing the pub would be a magnet for anti-sociality:

London Road has only just begun to establish itself as an acceptable area for families, locals and visitors with slightly less likelihood of intimidation by inebriated punters. There has been a massive input by the London Road Local Action Team, the police, the city council, and the Mary Portas project to transform an area that was woefully rundown and dangerous to a road we are all starting to feel proud of ... *Wetherspoons* has a bad reputation of encouraging excessive drinking with low cost alcohol and the effect on London Road would be detrimental. (Cited in an objection to planning application BH2015/00676, Wadsworth 2015)

Other new openings have proved similarly contentious: in the case of the aforementioned conversion of an old Whitstable cinema into a *Wetherspoons*, a local Labour councillor suggested naming the pub after the renowned actor Peter Cushing would be an insult 'if it becomes the place that some people fear it will' (cited in *Canterbury Times*, 27 May 2011). Objectors in this instance referred to the impact of a 'large pub offering cheap beer savagely affecting the already delicate economic balance of the town', predicting 'more anti-social behaviour, noise and disturbance, including fast food litter, bottles and cans being left outside private residences, and urination in the streets' (objection 25.10.2010, papers at licensing committee, Canterbury City Council 2010). Some even framed the issue as one of child protection, with 'a chain public house specializing in cut prices increasing the temptation for some families leading to more issues amongst their young children, who need safeguarding' (objection from St Alphage primary school cited in committee papers, ibid.). *Wetherspoons* pubs are effectively depicted as 'leaky' establishments, venues hoarding forms of drunken anti-sociality that threaten to spill over into the surrounding area, and contaminate the social body.

But why such concerns? Why is a pub, that is, from my own observations, a space where people read papers, do work, surf the Internet, watch TV, chat, flirt, and generally socialize, characterized by objectors as a repository of rowdy and anti-social behaviour? Clearly, these fears are not groundless, as any pub can attract anti-social elements, and be associated with late-night noise and nuisance. But the particular vehemence in which *Wetherspoons* appears to be held in certain quarters points to more fundamental anxieties relating to class and taste. In part, this is about snobbery. Like *McDonalds*, *Wetherspoons* is a chain that appears ubiquitous (even small towns like Loughborough and Dartford—both Portas pilot towns—boast a couple of *Wetherspoons* pubs, while in larger cities like Manchester and Nottingham, they are in double figures). Standardization and ubiquity are the enemies of the middle-class consumer, for whom a pub like *Wetherspoons* offers little opportunity to express distinction or cultural capital, for example, by choosing between a range of fine wines and local cask beers. Unlike many gastropubs on the High Street, the food comes on plates, not on slates, and most of it served with fries. Culturally, it takes its reference points from US sports bar culture more than 'sophisticated' European models of drinking and dining, following a model of provision whereby predictable food and drink is served in a setting which is comfortable and welcoming rather than one which emphasizes the distinction or status of the diners (cf. Kirkby 2008). Mark Brearley (2014: np) summarizes this attitude when he describes *Wetherspoons* as 'soulless, big, cheap city-centre drinking pits' (Fig. 5.1).

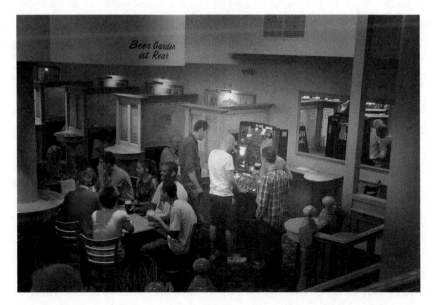

Fig. 5.1   A soulless drinking pit? 'The White Lion of Mortimer' Wetherspoons, Mitcham, London (photo: Chris Marchant, Flickr, used under a CCBY license)

So cultural snobbery might explain some of the negative reaction to *Wetherspoons'* High Street offer: even if we cannot be certain of the class background of those who object to their presence, there's a good chance most are the middle-class homeowners who are most motivated to protest against 'locally unwanted land uses' and get involved in NIMBY protest (Hubbard 2006; Matthews et al. 2014). Alan Warde et al. (1999) suggest that, in the contemporary consumer society, one does not show one's distinction by displaying overt cultural elitism. Rather, the sign of being a truly discerning and knowing consumer is to be culturally omnivorous and cosmopolitan, able to move between sites of 'low' and 'high' culture seamlessly, taking pleasure in both. Perhaps so. But there's something else that appears crucial here. *Wetherspoons* are, when compared with the other gastropub chains or independent pubs on our High Streets, cheap. Indeed, in the view of some financial analysts, they are 'unnecessarily cheap', the percentage of their range of food and drink falling into the heavily discounted bracket being much higher than it needs to be given the amount most are prepared to spend on a night out (Market Buzz 2015). And while the middle classes appear quite happy to search for a bargain in 'alternative' spaces of retail such as car boot fairs or jumble sales (Gregson et al. 2002), there appears to be something of a stigma associated with frequenting spaces which knowingly market themselves as discount or value chains. Why this might be is open to question. Perhaps it's because these sites are associated overwhelmingly with a white working class that's regularly depicted as the antithesis of a cosmopolitan consumer, being tied to tradition and little interested in new experiences and flavours.

The classed dimensions of the prejudice against *Wetherspoons* become clearer in ethnographic work that explores the consumption of nightlife. In William Haydock's (2014) study of drinking in Bournemouth, for example, *Wetherspoons* pubs were regularly referred to in derogatory terms by those who identified as more discerning, with a group of young investment bankers referring to the pub chain as a bit 'chavvy' and likely to be 'the type of place where unemployed people would be spending their green giros'. Such consumers sought to differentiate themselves from this clientele by emphasizing the idea that *Wetherspoons* consumers drink to get drunk, and exhibit a vulgar form of consumption based on facile or superficial pleasures rather than refined, deferred gratification (Haydock 2014). Given the body is a ubiquitous signifier of class (Skeggs 2005), it's apparent these assumptions are commonly read off and projected onto, 'chav' or 'townie' styles of dress which are dismissed as cheap and excessively showy. In contrast, valued spaces tend to be associated with alternative, individual fashions and sub-cultures. This is presented from the opposite perspective in the work of Anoop Nayak (2006), who presents a fascinating account of working-class masculinities in the North East in which chain pubs such as *Wetherspoons* allowed for the display of a 'real' white working-class identity, and attempts to recuperate the type of identities which predominated in the earlier, industrial era. For the young, working-class drinkers in his study, the ritual of going 'out on the town' to consume large amounts of alcohol was both affiliative and competitive: the ability to be able to 'handle' drink marking one out from one's peers. Alcohol consumption in such contexts is not necessarily about drinking to get drunk, but acquiring distinction. In previous generations, workingman's clubs and traditional pubs provided this type of space, their role now taken by *Wetherspoons* and the other chain pubs facilitating circuit drinking at minimal expenditure.

The use of the 'chav' shorthand to condemn spaces providing a space of identity and display for younger, working-class consumers—who, Nayak (2006: 821) suggests, have limited resource typically 'hard won through part-time work in the service sector employed at supermarkets, sports shops, petrol stations, record stores and cafés'—is telling. The 'chav' stereotype, as Owen Jones (2012) and others have argued, equates this lack of affluence with fecklessness and violence. In a nighttime economy where excessive or binge consumption of alcohol is associated with violence, it's cheap alcohol that's regarded with particular suspicion, and its consumers vilified. In this context, Conservative politicians have proposed a minimum unit price for alcohol as a potential solution to the problems of anti-sociality in the nighttime economy, something that would obviously have a disproportionate impact on poorer and heavier drinkers. Whether this would discourage such groups from drinking as much is a moot point: the chairman of *Wetherspoons*, Tim Martin's blunt assessment being 'It's utter bollocks basically … the problem with Cameron and Osborne is they have not worked in a fucking pub' (quoted in Goodley 2012: 12).

But, is much of this anxiety about vertical drinking, discount pub chains misplaced? Fiona Measham and Kevin Brain (2005) think so, arguing that it's not only a working-class minority who are prone to over-consumption in the nighttime economy, with the majority of middle-class consumers also disregarding safe drinking limits (which stand at around six pints of beer or glasses of wine per week). Yet, despite this, and a steady fall in binge drinking since the early 2000s, the notion that 'binge and brawl' drinking cultures are the provenances of working-class consumers remains prevalent. In part, this is because the media seems to dwell on the spectacular and carnivalesque forms of consumption which are apparent on particular 'drinking streets', ignoring the drinking and drunkenness occurring in more 'refined' or reputable spaces (Roberts and Eldridge 2007). But this emphasis on working-class excess is not new. Ever since the nineteenth century, ethnographers and media commentators alike have described nightlife as a site where 'unassimilated immigrants, a recalcitrant working class, new political movements, sexual deviants, and wayward youth subcultures' are seduced and 'demoralized' by commer-cialized sites of alcoholic pleasure and leisure (Mattson 2007: 76). In this sense, the fact the British High Street at night is now routinely associated with vulgar, debased and working-class drinking practices echoes many recurrent themes in the histories of drinking and drunkenness, giving them new life through a visceral language that evinces disgust reactions. In the words of Phil Hadfield et al. (2001: 300), the stereotyped 'Mass Volume Vertical Drinker' has assaulted the concept of the 24-hour city, with all its good intentions, 'leaving it for dead in streets splattered with blood, vomit, urine and the sodden remains of takeaways'.

Remoralizing the Night

Fuelled by images of 'continental' 'café culture', licensing policy in the 1990s succeeded in transforming the nighttime economy of British towns and cities. But, as we have seen, it did so at a cost. The resulting nighttime economy of alcohol-soaked 'drinkatainment' (Bell and Binnie 2005) has then been viewed as highly ambivalent, 'simultaneously conflictual and segregated, commodified and sanitized, saturated by both emotion (enhanced through alcohol, drugs, dance, sex, encounter) and rational elements (planning, surveillance and policing)' (Jayne et al. 2008: 88). In the eyes of policy-makers, the balance is often tipped towards the former, with the nighttime city requiring urgent attention in cases where it has proved most attractive to younger working-class drinkers to the detriment of other users and uses. In this respect, the rhetoric of some policy-makers and advisors is often blatant about the need to attract wealthier consumers back to the High Street at night. For example, ongoing plans to improve the quality of Bournemouth's nighttime 'offer' are predicated on the idea that the town needs more middle and upper class ('creative') consumers, and a different mix of venues in a town currently dominated by cheaper, chain pubs:

> The right type, not just any type, of after dark culture is vital … This report identifies the "cosmo-bar" as the type of place that the town centre requires more of if it's to be able to attract and retain more creative people. Without this diversification, the town will not fully benefit from a social and creative mix of people during the night-time … The lesson here for Bournemouth is that an active intervention in the town's evening and night-time economy to deliver a more diverse and welcoming place supports a message that the town is a creative and inclusive place. This is a vital message that inwards investors, entrepreneurs and job creators need to hear. This active intervention must be a partnership between the public, private and third sectors to have a real and meaningful effect. (Feria Urbanism for Bournemouth Town Watch Partnership 2012: 19)

In this report, the term 'cosmo-bar' is used to refer to a venue which eschews vertical drinking and discount alcohol in favour of a 'mixed' economy of eating, drinking and live entertainment. But more than this, the notion of 'cosmopolitanism' seems to signal an intent to steer the town away from the 'stag and hen' party crowd, which the media suggests is overwhelmingly catered for by the town's 50 or so bars and clubs. William Haydock (2014: 178) argues such visions make a clear connection between a particular mode of alcohol consumption and the presence of knowing, middle-class consumers, with the latter assumed to exert a civilizing influence on the town, 'as wealth is associated with the broader cultural attributes of these "better people"'.

However, efforts such as these to change the character of night-time economies are seldom couched in an explicit language of social improvement, being more normally justified in terms of community safety. Such policies take a number of forms, but in most cases are said to be reacting to perceived urban disorder (Hadfield 2014). Here, the use of licensing and planning law is certainly significant. Although the 2003 Licensing Act ushered in a more liberal attitude towards licensed premises, in recent years licensing committees have, in general, been more willing to withdraw licences from premises associated with anti-social behaviour, and have also refused licences in areas 'saturated' with drinking establishments. How this is determined is a matter of subjective judgement, and can vary from local authority to local authority, but many have now designated particular streets or neighbourhoods as 'saturation areas' for the purposes of alcohol licensing. While this option was always available to local authorities under the 2003 Licensing Act, initially it was not widely used. However, by 2014, there were some 208 of these (increased from 160 in 2012). While a local authority is obliged to consider each new application for a premises licence in a saturation area on its merits, government advice stipulates that if there's any objection made there should be an assumption against granting a licence unless the applicant can prove there will be no adverse cumulative impact. This relates to off-licenses (many of which sell beer and wine both day and night) as well as pubs and clubs. In part, this is a measure taken to discourage the practices of preloading or side-loading apparently rife in some spaces of nightlife (whereby 'circuit drinkers' will buy alcohol cheaply from off-licenses and consume it on the street before, or between, visits to bars). This has sometimes even extended to banning in-town supermarkets from selling alcohol: in Edinburgh, for example, some *Sainsburys Local* and *Tesco Metro* superstores have been forbidden from selling alcohol (or having strict limits placed on the amount of shelf-space devoted to beer, wine and spirits). Local authority licensing policies can also designate DPPOs (Designated Public Place Orders) or controlled drinking zones which give the police the power to prevent individuals consuming alcohol in stipulated public places if they are causing a nuisance (Jayne et al. 2011).

Policing is clearly significant here, as all local authorities are obliged to consult the police on all licence applications, and their objections carry much weight. Moreover, policing can enact forms of territoriality which subject particular communities and populations to scrutiny, not so much reacting to criminality but pre-empting it through visible 'reassurance policing' (Beckett and Herbert 2008). Eradicating street drinking can be a particular focus, irrespective of whether the drinking is problematic or actually causing nuisance. But given the cuts faced by the police, and the policy emphasis placed on partnership working, contemporary literatures on the policing of the nighttime economy speak of a 'surveillant assemblage' (Powell 2010: 208) involving 'an increasingly variegated mix of agencies including police, local authorities, health trusts, the licensed trade, security companies, residents groups, and charitable/voluntary agencies' (Hadfield et al. 2001: 466). In some cases, cooperative working is funded through the imposition of a late-night levy, which the coalition government introduced as a means of charging late-night businesses for the costs of policing the nighttime economy: local authorities can impose this charge on any business serving alcohol between midnight and six in the morning (exempting certain small businesses), splitting this revenue between the police (70%) and other agencies (30%). This means policing is not always by the police, with a plethora of third parties being significant in maintaining order on the streets: community support officers, street cleaners, local authority-funded taxi rank monitors, or even licensed taxi drivers (Shaw 2015). Here the lines between the voluntary sector and state-agencies are often blurred. For example, many local authorities provide funding to 'street pastors', with over 100 schemes thought to exist in the UK (Johns et al. 2009). These schemes are supposed to be non-interventionist, with pastors providing support to those who seek it in the nighttime economy by dispensing medical assistance, water, and, most notoriously, flip-flops for those trying to walk home drunkenly in high heels. However, research suggests their work 'not only reflects an ethics of care, ground rules for engagement and formal training but also personal views of who is, or is not, in need of help' (Middleton and Yarwood 2015: 511). While they are not part of formal Crime and Disorder partnerships, with their religious background preventing them from being closely associated with official state policy, street pastors can play a significant role in re-moralizing the night, viewing the city as 'a spiritual landscape' as they work alongside 'a wide range of secular partners in the contexts of their own (varied) Christian faith'.

Beyond this, it's evident that the remoralization of night is something being encouraged by businesses. Phil Hadfield (2014: 607) suggests that clubs, pubs and other nighttime venues can encourage or discourage particular types of consumption and consumer through a 'private governance of affect' whose role cannot be overstated. Technologies of surveillance are important here (especially CCTV, door supervisors and 'bouncers') but advertising, signage, décor, music and drinks menus can all be just as significant in terms of creating a particular 'vibe' or atmosphere. National initiatives have also been important here, such as the industry-led 'Best Bar None' scheme, which accredits those pubs that take measures to encourage responsible drinking. But rather than seeking to reform 'binge' drinkers, the aim here is more usually to attract a new, more discerning, customer base. Strategies of rebranding and renovation can be important for pubs or clubs adopting new business models based on rejecting high mass consumption in favour of a more selective offer. But this is something that can be enacted on a wider spatial scale too. For example, city centre management teams or those overseeing Business Improvement Districts can sometimes be charged with shifting the 'affective ambience' of entire entertainment districts. Robert Shaw (2015), for example, describes how Newcastle's 'Alive after Five' scheme has sought to attract a new and previously absent 'civilized' constituency to the city centre by appealing to those with interests in the arts, 'family activities', shopping and dining as well as the drinking for which Newcastle is famed. As in the Bournemouth plans described by William Haydock (2014), this is predicated on the idea that too much of the city is dominated by chain pubs and circuit drinkers, and that a more balanced and cosmopolitan vibe can be created by encouraging wealthier clientele and upmarket venues into areas that have become understood as 'drinking streets'.

Viewed in this light, it appears both the state and market are currently involved in concerted efforts to 'remoralize' the city at night via a range of post-disciplinary techniques focused on encouraging 'safer' and healthier modes of consumption. But how effective is this? Certainly, in terms of widening the cultural offer of the British High Street at night, it's been suggested there has been only limited progress outside of biggest cities. Alcohol consumption remains the lifeblood of most High Street and while this is routinely supplemented by takeaways, restaurants and night cafés, pubs remain the hubs around which nightlife revolves. Most cinemas and bingo halls are still out of town, and theatres limited to the larger provincial town and cities. Music venues too have decreased in number, seemingly part of an older, alternative mode of nightlife production 'displaced by a post-industrial mode of corporately-driven night-life production in the consumption-led city' (Chatterton and Hollands 2003: 78). So, while there's some evidence of changing attitudes to frequent drinking in the UK, with the recession no doubt having some influence, Fiona Measham and Karenza Moore's (2008) suggestion 'that drinkers display few signs of moving away from heavy sessional drinking, with the pursuit of the pharmacological pleasures of intoxication remaining a key priority for many consumers on a "big night out"' appears to hold good. Pubs and clubs remain the most profitable enterprises on the High Street at night.

However, there's evidence to suggest that the concerted attempt to create more 'civilized' nightlife is at least changing the way alcohol is consumed in many High Street premises. Increasingly, cheap keg lagers are shunned in favour of real cask ales, and cheap spirits are giving way to expensive 'craft gins' as drinkers are encouraged to be more discerning. 'Austerity nostalgia' is clearly influential here (Hatherley 2016), with pro-thrift agendas encouraging a burgeoning 'micro-industry' scene. These microbrewers and craft distillers trade on their homespun ethos and emphasize their pride in using traditional production methods, arguing it's worth spending a little more to support such 'authentic' production. At the same time, nostalgic staples such as pie and mash are to the fore, pork scratchings and kettle chips reinvented as retro gourmet snacks. Pub interiors have in some cases become matched to this post-war austerity aesthetic, with shabby chic furniture, 1950s festival of Britain tiling and typography to match. *The Meat and Barrel Craft Beer and Kitchen* on Southsea High Street (Palmerston Road) is a fairly typical example of the new breed. Open to the street, with large windows and a welcoming façade, it's fitted out with a mixture of distressed school-style chairs and battered but comfortable-looking brown button-leather sofas. It's decorated tastefully throughout: red brick exposed, industrial lighting, parquet floors and a funky illuminated sign proclaiming the venue as the 'Home of the Southsea Burger Club'. There's also white retro tiling behind the bar that puts into one's mind that the premises used to be a butchers or abattoir (though apparently that's not the case, despite the cow motif that is repeated throughout the premise). The bar itself is high and long and boasts a bewildering range—18 or so pumps—of cask ales and ciders, some from local Hampshire breweries, but also from further afield: Cornwall, Yorkshire, Wales and Lancashire, as well as lagers from Czechoslovakia and some US craft beers. The menu offers a range of beef, lamb and veggie burgers, all in toasted brioche buns (as befits the current fashion) for around £8-£10, and triple-cooked hand cut chips with barrel salt at £4 (they are half that or less in nearby chip shops down on the seafront).

While *The Meat and Barrel* appears unique, its brick and steelwork interior faithfully restored as a labour of love by two local entrepreneurs, it's becoming a fairly generic type of venue on contemporary High Streets, at least those in more affluent, whiter areas, which is certainly true of Southsea (overall, Portsmouth is 8% non-white according to the 2011 Census, but I do not see anyone in *The Meat and Barrel* who does not look thoroughly white and middle class on my visit). *Craft Burger*, Cromer, *Burger and Beers*, Edinburgh, *Burger Bros*, Broadstairs, *Firebrand*, Launceston, *Googies*, Folkestone, *Duke's*, Haggerston—and many, many others—have opened in the last few years providing a similar diet of craft beer and gourmet burgers, usually in a retro or shabby chic environment that matches the 'artisanal' vibe associated with craft production. There are even chains emerging to cash in on this fad—*Honest Burgers* has eight premises across London, expanding from its original 2011 Brixton base; *Meat* has outlets in Leeds, London and Brighton while the *Gourmet Burger Kitchen*, which first started trading in 2001, had over 60 restaurants in the UK by 2015. No doubt in a few short years the fashion for independently produced strong, hoppy beers and prime burgers will subside, but for now, this seems like a pretty profitable line of business, especially in those towns where there are large numbers of young professionals and bearded hipsters with high levels of disposable income. Tellingly, many of these new outlets have replaced previously struggling venues: according to the local newspaper, *The Meat and Barrel* replaced an 'unlamented' Chinese buffet restaurant when it opened in 2014.

So in many ways, the emergence of these types of upmarket, retro hipster bars on our High Streets seems to symbolize the rise of a new type of consumer experience in the evening economy. Gourmet burgers are not consumed as if one is at *McDonalds*, or the staple of the 1970s High Street, the *Wimpy* burger bar. Emphasis is on quality rather than quantity: the cut of beef, the provenance of the meat, the excellence of the bun and so on. The consumption of craft beers likewise requires a careful scrutiny of possible taste combinations, knowledge of different microbreweries, and a studied appreciation of labels that celebrate quirky cultural references. This is not about high consumption, bingeing or vertical drinking. Those who eat and drink at such venues, and who are prepared to pay a little more than they might do elsewhere for doing so, are exhibiting their social habitus (Bourdieu 1984), creating distinctions of class, gender and race in the process. There's a synergy between the goods on offer, the way they are advertised and the design of the premise. The sourcing of 'local' ingredients, the preference for limited run brews and the emphasis on the individual rather than the serially replicated all bequeath value on the act of consumption, and help create an 'authentic sense of self' for those seeking out these premises. As Vanessa Mathews and Roger Picton (2014: 341) argue, 'the discriminating craft brew consumer works as an agent of taste, perceptive of the symbolic value contained within each bottle and every pour'.

No wonder there's been little rhetoric of opposition to the emergence of such premises on our High Streets. As we have seen, nighttime businesses serving 'discount' alcohol are regarded with suspicion, but in contrast, there's little anxiety expressed about fashionable premises where it's assumed the clientele is interested in quality, not quantity. The fact that craft beers are generally higher alcohol content than the lagers, milds and bitters served in many chain pubs does not enter into things as it's assumed that the consumer of craft beers is more interested in drinking than getting drunk. The fact that microbrews are relatively expensive is in their favour in this regard, with 330 ml bottles of Punk IPA or Kernel Microbrew selling for more than the typical pint, favouring their adoption as the drink of choice by the knowing, middle class. Their price actually reinforces their perception of being authentic, a 'real' alternative to mass-produced lagers or flavoured vodkas, and middle-class consumers are often prepared to pay a little more for them. Perversely, the idea that ale was traditionally a working-class drink is also not forgotten, with local brewing's apparent 'resistance' to global corporate producers and national pub chains meaning there's little negative discourse about the price of microbrews, despite their popularity among the urban hipsters gentifying working-class cultures (see also Spracklen et al. 2013, on 'real ale'). Here, it's worth reiterating that hipsters are not necessarily counter-cultural, and are generally from wealthy rather than working-class backgrounds.

This targeting of a hip, knowing urbanite—or at least a more wealthy clientele—appears ubiquitous among new businesses on the British High Street. But it can take markedly different forms. In the fishing port of Whitstable, for example, two new pubs have opened since the arrival of *Wetherspoons* in 2012. But when *Black Dog* opened in 2013 and *Handsome Sams* in 2014, the type of opposition voiced against *Wetherspoons* was nowhere to be found, despite the fact that both new pubs were to specialize in the cask ales that *Wetherspoons* sell at a similarly competitive price. Both, instead, were discoursed as part of a new 'micropub' movement vaunted as 'restoring life' on the High Street: the former opened in a bankrupt antiques store, the latter in a vacant greengrocers. The micropub 'movement' is thought to have started in Kent in 2005 when a former butcher's shop in Herne (*The Butcher's Arms*) became the first self-styled micropub and set down a no-frills and nostalgic template focused on the consumption of traditional ales and bar snacks. By 2013, there were 50 micropubs, mainly in Kent, with the hundredth opening in December 2014, and 166 by the end of 2015, as the idea spread across the country. The names betray the fact that most have required planning permission to convert a previous retail use to a venue serving alcohol: the *Barber's Arms* in Wye, *The Old Post Office*, Warwick, *Cobblers*, Cinderford, *The Bake and Alehouse*, Westgate (in an old bakery), and *The Overdraft* (in an old bank), Southampton. All boast minimal décor with seating designed to encourage conversation between customers, most of it reclaimed school or factory furniture. The décor is typically spartan, exposed brickwork and bare bulbs (Fig. 5.2). Most serve basic bar snacks (but no meals), and there's a distinct absence of any music or electronic entertainment, with even mobile phone use being discouraged. Above all else, barrels or casks

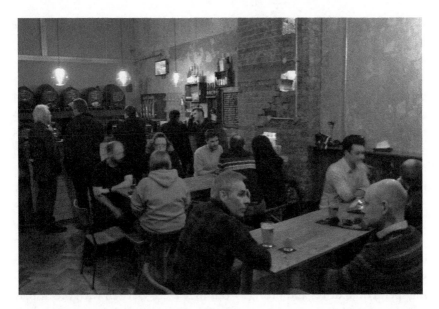

Fig. 5.2 The Overdraft micropub, in an old bank building, Shirley, Southampton (photo: author)

of beer are given prominence, with blackboards typically describing the origins, flavor, and alcohol content of individual beers. This focus on real ale (and very occasionally wine) gives such venues their *raison d'etre*, and also their favourable reputation with the local planners and licensing officers who seem willing to facilitate their opening even in locations where other pubs might be refused permission. Martyn Hillier, the owner of the *Butcher's Arms* at Herne and founder of the micropubs association gives a possible explanation. 'We don't sell lager … beer has more hops which have a soporific effect. No one gets drunk in my pub, they get sleepy', he argues, continuing 'The police have never been called to break up a fight at a micropub.' When I chat to the chief licensing officer who dealt with the pub's application, he confirms this stereotype, suggesting that local residents are not particularly worried about small pubs being set up by 'hobbyist' owners because there's a perception they will be frequented by an older, discerning clientele, not high-volume consumers. 'Local people think the pub's going to be opening late in the day and closing early', he says, continuing by suggesting that 'they don't realise that once a licence is granted they are potentially paving the way for a future owner to open that same premise later, and louder'.

Currently, however, the dominant image of a micropub is one of a community-minded premise grounded in 'traditional' British cultures of drinking rather than 'continental' café culture, and, perhaps unsurprisingly, it's one little opposed by local residents. Indeed, the micropub is regarded as a generally benevolent presence on High Streets at a time when other shops and businesses are closing (West 2014). Visiting such premises, one is struck that most have a mixed, but somewhat older and mainly male, clientele that may have been introduced to real ale in their working youth, but who are now drinking in micropubs to avoid engaging with the younger, poorer and working-class drinkers they might encounter in chain or tenanted pubs. It's worth noting here that these venues are not expensive—indeed, they are able to provide beer relatively cheaply by minimizing spend on fixtures and fittings—but they are associated with the display of cultural capital via a nostalgic disavowal of 'popular' culture and there are none of the brands familiar to those used to buying drinks from bargain booze outlet. Beers are discussed and sampled, not just drunk, and there's little to distract from that key activity. This is distinctly gendered: Thurnell-Read (2013: 3) reminds us 'drinking is evidently a terrain through which both normalised and problematic embodiments of masculinity are enacted and policed', continuing by arguing that 'in a general sense, those who drink alcohol in a sensible manner can distinguish themselves from those seen to lack control'. Those in micropubs conform to this ideal, their leisurely consumption showing they appreciate 'craft' brewing and are drinking to enjoy the beer, not simply to get drunk. The distinction made between pubs and micropubs then is not just one of scale, it's one of class and the search for a sense of identity in which one's social status can be connected both to what one drinks, and where (Järvinen et al. 2014).

This highlights a situation where cheap alcohol on the High Street is regularly condemned as a health risk, a cue to anti-sociality and an enticement to bingeing, but certain businesses offering cheap drinks are nonetheless encouraged, apparently because they offer a different *style* of drinking. This complex collision of culture and capital is important in the context of High Street gentrification given both the individual enthusiasts who invest 'sweat equity' in their microbusinesses and the corporations buying up cheap premises are implicated in changing patterns of consumption that ultimately make areas culturally unattractive and unaffordable to working-class residents. Despite the claim that pubs and cafés are somehow outside these processes (see Ernst and Doucet 2014), the truth is that nightlife spaces are key drivers of gentrification, with transition in the nighttime and evening economy being highly symbolic of class-transition (as Jackson and Benson 2014 note when they describe the importance of pubs to gentrification in areas of Peckham and Dulwich). Indeed, the pub is a key space in gentrification debates, given, it often embodies a resistance to change (e.g., by emphasizing local traditions) while simultaneously pacifying that resistance through a retro-chic commodification of working-class identities (Mathews and Picton 2014).

Whatever, a number of contemporary commentators hypothesize that recent efforts to produce a more civilized nighttime economy, where micropubs are favoured over 'drinking barns' and craft beer over lager and shots, can only result in a gentrification of the night. Put simply, people are being encouraged to spend more but consume less, meaning that those used to spending little are finding their hold on the High Street after dark increasingly precarious. Indeed, this gentrification is marginalizing both the traditional working-class pubs that were rendered surplus to requirements in the post-industrial corporate city (Chatterton and Hollands 2003), as well as the corporatized spaces of mass alcohol consumption that came to characterize many post-industrial city centres. This process of nighttime gentrification is making it harder for more marginal and poorer social groups to have any sort of presence in the city at night. This is akin to the process noted by Laam Hae (2011) (amongst others) in the USA, where gentrification has often relied upon a discoursing of difference and the identification of specific neighbourhoods as having a vibrant nightlife offer which is the antithesis of that evident on the out-of-town leisure 'strip'. As she argues:

> Nightlife establishments often constitute an important foundation for the rekindling of depressed property markets in derelict neighbourhoods by helping to generate an atmosphere of lively urban sociality. In particular, nightlife establishments associated with inner-city sub-cultures, such as underground

music/performance clubs, add a particular aura to the neighbourhoods, often leading to 'hipster gentrification'. However, it has simultaneously been observed that, once gentrification settles in, nightlife businesses have been pushed out of the very neighbourhoods that they helped to market as interesting to outsiders. (Hae 2013: 3450)

In a UK context, Deborah Talbot (2011) argues the combined assault of commercialism, social order concerns and regulatory practice has long closed down the experimental possibilities of nightlife and alternative culture in the UK, particularly that associated with black and ethnic minority groups (given the suspicion expressed towards venues offering grime, garage, reggae or R&B). Even though there may be a reaction to the more branded and larger chains on our High Streets, this is apparently not one providing increased opportunity to such groups, nor to working-class consumers. For the moment, *Wetherspoons* and other venues offering relatively cheap nighttime entertainment and leisure remain on the High Street—even in Southsea—but the general push to remoralize the night, and encourage a more 'balanced' High Street, only appears to be heading in one direction: a segregation of the nighttime on class lines that will increasingly push the poorer in society away from the High Street and back into their own homes.

References

Allen, J., Edmonds, S., Patterson, A., & Smith, D. (2005). *Policing and the criminal justice system-public confidence and perceptions: Findings from the 2003/04 British Crime Survey*. London, UK: Home Office.

Andrews, D., & Turner, S. (2012). Is the pub still the hub? *International Journal of Contemporary Hospitality Management, 24*(4), 542–552.

Beaumont, M. (2015). *Nightwalking: A nocturnal history of London*. Verso Books.

Beckett, K., & Herbert, S. (2008). Dealing with disorder: Social control in the post-industrial city. *Theoretical Criminology, 12*(1), 5–30.

Bell, D., & Binnie, J. (2005). What's eating Manchester? Gastro-culture and urban regeneration. *Architectural Design, 75*(3), 78–85.

Bourdieu, P. (1984). *Distinction: A social critique of the judgment of taste.* Cambridge: Harvard University Press.

Brearley, M. (2014). Wetherspoons pubs: Soulless drinking pits or mainstay of the High Street? The *Guardian*, 4 April, http://www.theguardian.com/lifeand-style/wordofmouth/2014/apr/04/wetherspoon-pubs-real-ale-beer-high-street

Brierley-Jones, L., Ling, J., McCabe, K. E., Wilson, G. B., Crosland, A., Kaner, E. F., et al. (2014). Habitus of home and traditional drinking: A qualitative analysis of reported middle-class alcohol use. *Sociology of Health & Illness, 36*(7), 1054–1076.

Brooks, O. (2014). Interpreting young women's accounts of drink spiking: The need for a gendered understanding of the fear and reality of sexual violence. *Sociology, 48*(2), 300–316.

Bromley, R., Thomas, C., & Millie, A. (2000). Exploring safety concerns in the night-time city: Revitalising the evening economy. *Town Planning Review, 71*(1), 71.

Burgess, A., Donovan, P., & Moore, S. E. (2009). Embodying uncertainty? Understanding heightened risk perception of drink 'spiking'. *British Journal of Criminology, 49*(6), 848–862.

Campbell, E. (2012). Transgression, affect and performance choreographing a politics of urban space. *British Journal of Criminology, 53*(1), 18–40.

Canterbury City Council. (2010). Minutes of Licensing Sub-Committee. 7 December, Guildhall, Canterbury.

Chatterton, P., & Hollands, R. (2003). *Urban nightscapes: Youth cultures, pleasure spaces and corporate power.* London: Routledge.

Department of Communities and Local Government (DCLG) (2012). *Reimagining urban spaces to revitalize our High Streets.* London: DCLG.

Ernst, O., & Doucet, B. (2014). A window on the (changing) neighbourhood: The role of pubs in the contested spaces of gentrification. *Tijdschrift voor Economische en Sociale Geografie, 105*(2), 189–205.

Feria Urbanism for Bournemouth Town Watch Partnership (2012). *Bournemouth by night: Final report.* Bournemouth Borough Council: Bournemouth.

Finney, A. (2004). Violence in the night-time economy: Key findings from the research. Home Office Research Findings 214. London: Home Office.

Florida, R. (2002). *The rise of the creative class.* New York: Basic Books.

Goodley, S. (2012). Drinks industry refuses to swallow government line on alcohol pricing. The Observer, Sunday 4 November.

Gregson, N., Crewe, L., & Brooks, K. (2002). Shopping, space, and practice. *Environment and Planning (D)—Society and Space, 20*(5), 597–618.

Habermas, J. (1991). *The structural transformation of the public sphere: An inquiry into a category of bourgeois society*. Boston: MIT Press.

Hadfield, P. (2006). *Bar wars: Contesting the night in contemporary British cities*. Oxford: Oxford University Press.

Hadfield, P. (2014). The night-time city. Four modes of exclusion: Reflections on the Urban Studies special collection. *Urban Studies, 52*(3), 606–616.

Hadfield, P., Lister, S., Hobbs, D., & Winlow, S. (2001). The "24-hour city"— Condition critical. *Town and Country Planning., 70*, 300–302.

Hae, L. (2011). Dilemmas of the nightlife fix. *Urban Studies, 48*(16), 3449–3465.

Hatherley, O. (2016). *The Ministry of Nostalgia*. London: Verso.

Haydock, W. (2014). The 'civilising' effect of a 'balanced' night-time economy for 'better people': Class and the cosmopolitan limit in the consumption and regulation of alcohol in Bournemouth. *Journal of Policy Research in Tourism, Leisure and Events, 6*(2), 172–185.

Hayward, K., & Hobbs, D. (2007). Beyond the binge in 'booze Britain': Market-led liminalization and the spectacle of binge drinking. *The British Journal of Sociology, 58*(3), 437–456.

Holloway, S. L., Jayne, M., & Valentine, G. (2008). 'Sainsbury's is my local': English alcohol policy, domestic drinking practices and the meaning of home. *Transactions of the Institute of British Geographers, 33*(4), 532–547.

Hubbard, P. (2003). Fear and loathing at the multiplex: Everyday anxiety in the post-industrial city. *Capital & Class, 27*(2), 51–75.

Hubbard, P. (2006). *Key ideas in Geography—The City*. London: Routledge.

Hubbard, P. (2013). Carnage! Coming to a town near you? Nightlife, uncivilised behaviour and the carnivalesque body. *Leisure Studies, 32*(3), 265–282.

Jackson, E., & Benson, M. (2014). Neither 'deepest, darkest Peckham' nor 'run-of-the-mill' East Dulwich: The middle classes and their 'others' in an inner-London neighbourhood. *International Journal of Urban and Regional Research, 38*(4), 1195–1210.

Jayne, M., Valentine, G., & Holloway, S. L. (2011). *Alcohol, drinking, drunkeness: (dis)orderly spaces*. Farnham: Ashgate.

Jayne, M., Valentine, G., & Holloway, S. L. (2008). Fluid boundaries—'British' binge drinking and 'European' civility: Alcohol and the production and consumption of public space. *Space and Polity, 12*(1), 81–100.

Johns, N., Squire, G., & Barton, A. (2009). Street pastors: From crime prevention to re-moralisation? *British Society of Criminology online journal, 9*, 39–56.

Jones, O. (2012). *Chavs: The demonization of the working class*. London: Verso.

Kirkby, D. (2008). "From Wharfie Haunt to Foodie Haven": Modernity and law in the transformation of the Australian working-class pub. *Food, Culture & Society, 11*(1), 29–48.

Landry, C., & Bianchini, F. (1995). *The creative city*. London: Demos.

Lovatt, A., & O'Connor, J. (1995). Cities and the night-time economy. *Planning Practice and Research, 10*(2), 127–134.

Market Buzz (2015) Wetherspoon's beer unnecessarily cheap, 21 January. http://www.sharecast.com/news/wetherspoon-s-beer-unnecessarily-cheap/22409691.html

Mathews, V., & Picton, R. M. (2014). Intoxifying gentrification: Brew pubs and the geography of post-industrial heritage. *Urban Geography, 35*(3), 337–356.

Matthews, P., Bramley, G., & Hastings, A. (2014). Homo-economicus in a Big Society: Understanding middle-class activism and NIMBYism towards new housing developments. *Housing, Theory and Society, 32*(1), 54–72.

Mattson, G. (2007). Urban ethnography's "saloon problem" and its challenge to public sociology. *City & Community, 6*(2), 75–94.

Measham, F., & Brain, K. (2005). 'Binge' drinking, British alcohol policy and the new culture of intoxication. *Crime, Media, Culture, 1*(3), 262–283.

Measham, F., & Moore, K. (2008). The criminalisation of intoxication. In P. Squires (Ed.), *ASBO Nation: The criminalisation of nuisance*. Bristol: Policy Press.

Middleton, J., & Yarwood, R. (2015). 'Christians, out here?' Encountering Street-Pastors in the post-secular spaces of the UK's night-time economy. *Urban Studies, 52*(3), 501–516.

Monkkonen, E. H. (1981). A disorderly people? Urban order in the nineteenth and twentieth centuries. *The Journal of American History, 68*(3), 539–559.

Nayak, A. (2006). Displaced masculinities: Chavs, youth and class in the post-industrial city. *Sociology, 40*(5), 813–831.

Nead, L. (2000). *Victorian Babylon: People, streets, and images in nineteenth-century*. London: Yale University Press.

Norman, W. (2011). *Rough Nights: The growing dangers of working at night*. London: Young Foundation.

Powell, R. (2010). Spaces of informalisation: Playscapes, power and the governance of behaviour. *Space and Polity, 14*(2), 189–206.

Roberts, M. (2004). *Good practice in managing the evening and late night economy: A literature review from an environmental perspective*. London: Office of the Deputy Prime Minister.

Roberts, M., & Eldridge, A. (2007). Quieter, safer, cheaper: Planning for a more inclusive evening and night-time economy. *Planning, Practice & Research, 22*(2), 253–266.

Schivelbusch, W. (1988). *Disenchanted night: The industrialization of light in the nineteenth century.* Berkeley: University of California Press.

Schlör, J. (1998). *Nights in the big city: Paris, Berlin, London 1840–1930.* London: Reaktion Books.

Sharpe, W. (2008). *New York nocturne: The city after dark in literature, painting, and photography, 1850–1950.* Princeton, NJ: Princeton University Press.

Shaw, R. (2015). 'Alive after five': Constructing the neoliberal night in Newcastle upon Tyne. *Urban Studies, 52*(3), 456–470.

Skeggs, B. (2005). The making of class and gender through visualizing moral subject formation. *Body, Culture and Society, 39*(5), 965–982.

Spracklen, K., Laurencic, J., & Kenyon, A. (2013). 'Mine's a Pint of Bitter': Performativity, gender, class and representations of authenticity in real-ale tourism. *Tourist Studies, 13*(3), 304–321.

Talbot, D. (2011). The juridification of nightlife and alternative culture: Two UK case studies. *International Journal of Cultural Policy, 17*(1), 81–93.

Thurnell-Read, T. (2013). 'Yobs' and 'Snobs': Embodying drink and the problematic male drinking body. *Sociological Research Online, 18*(2), 3.

Warde, A., Martens, L., & Olsen, W. (1999). Consumption and the problem of variety: Cultural omnivorousness, social distinction and dining out. *Sociology, 33*(1), 105–127.

West, B. (2014). Community fixers? The mighty rise of the micropub. The New Statesman, 18 September, http://www.newstatesman.com/culture/2014/09/community-fixers-mighty-rise-micropub

Wodsworth, J. (2015). Wetherspoons refusal followed scores of objections. *Brighton & Hove News*, 1 June, p. 7.

Zukin, S. (1998). Urban lifestyles: Diversity and standardisation in spaces of consumption. *Urban Studies, 35*(5-6), 825–839.

6

Sexing It Up

In 2013, a new store opened in Poole, on the English south coast, in an area of the High Street described in the local press as 'a run-down part of town known for empty units, charity shops and cut price retailers' (Astrup 2013: np). This new opening was seemingly good news in a town centre struggling in times of recession, and which had applied—albeit unsuccessfully—to be one of Mary Portas' pilot town projects. Given that a report on the town's retail health stressed the vacancy rate was above the national average, leaving areas appearing 'rather tired and neglected in places' (Peter Brett Associates 2013), the fact that the new premises owner had spent £100,000 ensuring the shop would be 'the best looking in Poole' was surely to be welcomed. But the store in question—*Purrfectly Discreet*—was one specializing in lingerie, sex toys and other 'adult products', the windows obscuring the interior of the store hosting two large images of female models in lingerie. The owner of a schoolwear shop opposite appeared especially angry, arguing 'families will think twice before coming along here … when people ask for directions to the schoolwear shop I don't think I'm going to be happy to say go along to the sex shop and cross the road'. Jonathan Sibbett, chairman of Poole Town Centre Management Board, also went on record to state

© The Editor(s) (if applicable) and The Author(s) 2017
P. Hubbard, *The Battle for the High Street*,
DOI 10.1057/978-1-137-52153-8_6

the new shop was 'detrimental' to their plans to enhance the appeal of the High Street, suggesting 'this shop will not fit in with the mix of current retailers and will therefore affect the achievement of our aims' (cited in Astrup, ibid.). Some other residents were more blunt in their assessment:

> A sex shop would deteriorate this delicate economic area of Poole … why would they want to put a sordid shop slap bang in the middle of the High Street near community centres, youth groups, toddler crèches, and other sensitive community projects where young and vulnerable people visit on a regular basis. I certainly will not be visiting the High Street if the shop is granted a licence. (Objection considered at Poole Licensing Subcommittee, 10th July 2013)

This type of local furor around the opening of sex shops is not atypical, and in many instances, opposition has been sufficient to convince local authorities that granting a licence for a sex shop would be inappropriate as it might 'lower the tone' of a given locality. However, in the case of *Purrfectly Discreet*, the shop ultimately obtained a licence for the sale of 'restricted' products and DVDs, albeit the licensing authority required the frosting of the windows 'to protect children and vulnerable people', demanding the removal of the photos of models in lingerie.

This debate about the presence of sex retailers on the High Street matters because, whichever way you look at it, sex sells. Indeed, it's often described as recession-proof. In the recent economic downturn, online sex retailers have reported recorded profits, and in the more profitable and high-end corners of the metropolis, designer boutiques like *Agent Provocateur* and *Coco De Mer* have maintained a steady trade selling burlesque-style lingerie and high-end sex toys (e.g. balcony bras for £110, a Soiree patent leather cat whip for £325, and an 18 karat gold-plated vibrator for an eye-watering £12,000). Yet, there are many who have gone on record to suggest the British High Street is shamed by sex retailing, and a similarly vocal contingent arguing some High Streets have been coarsened by the emergence of 'lap dance' clubs offering sexual entertainment to adult audiences (Hubbard 2009). Local resident groups, business representatives and religious groups alike frequently petition local authorities with the intention of preventing such premises opening, while at a national level, these protests have coalesced into successful campaigns lobbying for new legislation allowing for tighter control of such premises. As we will see, sex establishments are an embattled space on the contemporary British High Street, their opening often discouraged by punitively high licensing fees and local authority policies which preclude their opening in 'inappropriate localities' (which in practice can mean anywhere vaguely close to a school, place of worship, or other 'communal facility'). This means lap dance clubs are slowly disappearing, while sex shops are increasingly located on industrial estates where there's no residential community to oppose them.

The fact that regulatory policies are pushing sex establishments off local shopping streets seemingly contradicts those national policies arguing for High Street renewal. In an era when retail confidence in the High Street has been sorely tested, and vacancies abound, sex shops and sex entertainment venues add variation to many High Streets, potentially attracting new consumers. Opponents would, of course, argue these are the 'wrong sort' of consumers, describing these as abject, dirty, or perverted. In contrast, owners are at pains to stress that their establishments are now frequented by men, women and couples (both straight and gay) and that their clientele is not the 'dirty mac brigade' of yesteryear, but a wider demographic. The success of erotic novel *Fifty Shades of Grey* in bringing 'kink' to the mainstream has certainly been a factor here, though the putative 'normalization' of sexual consumption arguably has wider and more complex roots, with the proliferation of sexual content on the internet no doubt significant. In this light, it appears somewhat odd that sex establishments themselves remain vilified in many quarters, with the only 'sex' premises appearing widely accepted on the High Street being those female-friendly outlets—particularly *Ann Summers*—which are variously referred to as 'adult sexuality boutiques' (Edwards 2010: 135) or 'erotic boutiques' (Smith 2007: 167) rather than sex shops per se. Amber Martin (2013: 81) argues that such erotic boutiques are 'essentially free to locate in any geographical location with no form of regulation' because they do not sell the type of restricted products which require a sex shop licence, noting that 'it's not uncommon for erotic boutiques to be located next to toy shops' or other outlets targeting children. A key question then is, why these particular stores are accepted on the High Street while other sex establishments are condemned for 'lowering the tone'. Is this simply because they do not sell the R18 Pornographic videos that would necessitate their licensing as a sex shop? Or is it related to the fact that these light, open and stylish stores are explicitly marketed to women, and hence assuage some of the traditional British anxieties that exist concerning the relations of class, morality and sex?

Just Another Shop? Sex Retailing on the High Street

Histories of pornography suggest that objects and media designed to sexually arouse have always been available to those who knew where to find them, albeit this access was often highly gendered, with men generally determined to prevent women, children and those with 'insufficiently socialized sensibilities' from consuming sexual images and content (Hunter et al. 1993: 65). Indeed, it was as recently as the 1970s that the 'sex shop' emerged in Britain as a recognizable retail form that clearly indicated its purpose to all (Coulmont and Hubbard 2010). In effect, such shops brought together various items previously sold elsewhere (i.e. through specialist bookshops, in pharmacies, lingerie shops or by specialist mail order), offering them in an environment that left little ambiguity as to their sexual nature. Emerging in the wake of the 1960s 'sexual revolution', such spaces attracted considerable press interest, much of it discussing whether the widespread consumption of sexually explicit materials was morally corrosive, and potentially undermining the 'family values' on which the post-war prosperity of Britain had seemingly been founded. While much of this discussion focused on Soho—London's de facto red light district—the opening of sex shops in the provinces also excited much discussion, and no little opposition. The proliferation of David Gold's *Private Shops* in the 1970s and 1980s was a case in point, with controversial openings in Portsmouth, Plymouth and Cheltenham (amongst others) leaving the local authorities involved distraught they had no means to control what were perfectly legal businesses given their content rarely exceeded the thresholds of decency enshrined in the *Obscene Publications Acts* of 1959 and 1964 (Manchester 1990).

The underlying causes of anxiety about sex shops are open to multiple conjectures, but appear to relate to modern assumptions that sex is something that can be enjoyed in the private/personal sphere, but when visible in the public realm is obscene or simply disgusting. Pornography, for example, is widely consumed in private, but its display and sale in the relatively open public space of a shop is something that transgresses the boundaries deemed necessary to maintain social and moral order given this involves a commercial transaction between strangers rather than one occurring in the private sphere of intimate relations. Those who work in such stores hence perform a form of 'dirty work' (Tyler 2011), while customers also have to negotiate abject identities. As outlined in French feminist psychoanalyst Julia Kristeva's (1982) influential *Powers of Horror*, abjection is the process in which the boundary between Self and Other becomes blurred, and in which the individual seeks to cast off or repel that which disturbs the distinction between their body's inside and the world outside. The abject body is one that leaks wastes and fluids, violates its own borders and does not conform to social standards of cleanliness or propriety (Shildrick 1997). Disgust is the primary embodied reaction to encountering such bodies—or even representations of such bodies—in public, with geographer David Sibley (1995) consequently arguing the urge to exclude the abject from one's proximity is perfectly explicable given our desire to maintain bodily cleanliness and purity. Bad objects and bad bodies are thus distanced through processes designed to purify or sanitize: historically, 'polluting' materials and populations have been segregated from more respectable, cleaner neighbourhoods, and pushed towards areas which become known as areas of 'ill repute' (Hubbard 2013). This can involve individual community actions or protests intended to remove commercial sex from particular localities, but more frequently involves the deployment of techniques of governmentality as enacted by municipal bureaucrats and officials (such as planners, licensing officers and environmental health inspectors). As a consequence, sex shops have traditionally been located in non-residential areas and typically run-down inner city districts rather than prominent High Streets. The nature of these spaces reaffirms dominant myths about sex shops: as Paul Maginn and Christine Steinmitz (2014: 264) argue, 'the sexualized nature of the city is reflected symbolically, physically, culturally and commercially in our sociological and geographical imaginations', with the place and space of sex shops seen to reflect their somewhat 'immoral' nature.

Such perspectives on the moral geography of sex shops have been explored by several commentators engaging with theories of spatial governmentality that, via Michel Foucault, focus on the ways populations are managed through a deliberative manipulation of urban space. In focusing on different *techne*—e.g. licensing, planning, judiciary—used by local authorities and the state to emplace commercial sex within existing property rights regimes, studies such as those by Emily Van der Meulen and Mariana Valverde (2013) or Mary Laing (2012) have shown the regulation of commercial sex in the city needs to be understood as implicated in the wider biopolitics central to liberal forms of governmentality (Legg 2005). Governmentality refers here to a 'mentality of government', both in the sense of how the government thinks about its governed citizens and how those citizens think about themselves, while *techne* refers to modes of government intervention into the reality of the lived urban population (Foucault 1991). Here, instruments such as development control are used to organize and to establish rules concerning the effective use of urban space, approving some businesses but refusing others. These decisions about which businesses 'belong' in different urban spaces—such as High Streets—are hence 'authorized' by the bodies charged with managing common interests on behalf of the municipality (e.g. licensing committees, planning committees).

Such ideas help explain the 'traditional' geography of sex shops in Britain, and pornography more generally: the chief role of the state in relation to pornography has not been to ban it outright, but ensure it's not visible in the neighbourhoods where it's most likely to prompt disgust. This logic informed the system of sex shop licensing introduced through the provisions of sections 2 and 3 of the *Local Government (Miscellaneous Provisions) Act 1982*, which was a response to the lobbying of those local authorities that considered they needed stronger powers to shape the location and visibility of sex shops in the city. Although this Act allowed local authorities little power to determine what was sold in sex shops, it allowed them to prohibit the display of products in shop windows, ban access to under-18s, and restrict opening hours (typically to daytime only). The new Act also allowed licence refusal on a number of grounds, such as the 'character of the applicant' or the unsuitability of the location. In relation to the latter, local authorities were encouraged to consider the character of the 'relevant locality' and the uses to which any premises in the vicinity were put. Refusal of a sex shop licence was made possible if 'the number of sex establishments in the relevant locality at the time the application is made is equal to or exceeds the number which the authority consider is appropriate for the locality', with the local authority at liberty to decide none may be appropriate. Here, test cases suggest definitions of 'the relevant locality' are a matter to be decided according to the circumstances of an application, leaving local authorities with considerable discretion to not to grant a licence if they decide the location is inappropriate: annual renewal also gives them leeway to refuse renewal if they decide that material changes to an area mean an existing sex shop is no longer appropriate in a given location (Manchester 1990).

The upshot of this mode of regulation was that while many towns and cities had a licensed sex shop by the 1990s, the majority of these were located away from the High Street, often in the inner city or marginal retail locations. Moreover, because of the enforced obscuring of the interior from the street, these appeared 'oases of ugliness' whose blacked-out windows created a fear of what lurked within, especially for female consumers (Tyler 2012). Reflecting on this, Fran Carter suggests that there's been a persistent gendering of the sex shop in Britain:

> Visually, the image of the traditional sex shop looms large in the collective female imagination, its stereotypical location on a dingy side alley in an area characterized by its bookmakers, barber shops and tagareen [*junk*] stores, the sweetly cloying smell of years of furtive urination around a darkened doorway, the grimy blacked-out windows with their stuttering neon signs—the women I interviewed uniformly constructed the male sex shop using the terms 'seedy', 'sordid' or 'sleazy'. (Carter 2014: 101)

When 'combined with the notion that male sexuality is exploitative and dark', the sex shop symbolized 'a place abandoned to sleaze and inadequacy' (Smith 2007: 169). In Clarissa Smith's (2007) view, this encouraged a furtive and anonymous consumption of pornography and reproduced sex shops as solely male preserves.

However, this began to change with the emergence of stores marketing sex-related products primarily to women. *Ann Summers* was the main pioneer here, growing from a solitary (male-run) shop in the 1970s to 40 outlets in 1999 and over 140 in 2015 across Britain and Ireland (Fig. 6.1). This success has been built on a clear strategy of steering the store away from male fantasies of femininity and towards particular ideas of how women want to look and feel, with stores being marketed at, staffed by and owned by women. An important part of this 'feminisation' has been the development of strong brand identity that has been mirrored in the store's design:

> The female orientation of the store is expressed in the shop space by the emphatic use of the colour pink throughout the shop's interior and exterior, which is also seen in other erotic boutiques … In Western society the colour pink is symbolically associated with 'romance and femininity' and

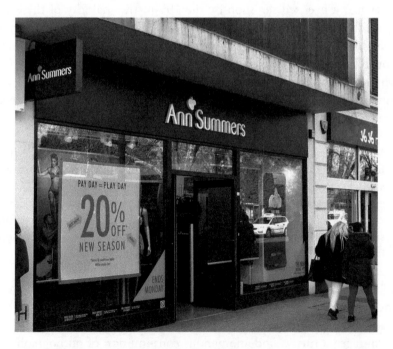

Fig. 6.1 Sex on the High Street—Ann Summers shop, Southampton (photo: author)

the female gender, while pale pastel pinks are commonly 'associated with little girls' … The use of pink throughout the shop draws on the stereotypical association with infantilized femininity. In addition, the pink décor produces an affective sensory experience of being cocooned in a female-friendly 'safe-space'. (Martin 2013: 60)

In Evans et al.'s (2010: 219) study of women's consumption of sex shops, the internal appearance of *Ann Summers* was affirmatively interpreted by the women they interviewed as 'addressing female consumers in highly autoerotic and individualistic ways'. This strong feminine aesthetic is a far cry from the traditional backstreet sex shop, with the stores presenting themselves as 'gynocentric playspaces' (Malina and Schmidt 1997: 167): their advertising has likewise targeted 'real' women, using non-professional models, and sought to capitalize on the publicity given to the hedonistic forms of women's sexual agency presented in *Sex and The City*, *50 Shades of Grey*, *Secret Diary of a Call Girl* and other popular representations of feminine sexuality. The chain has also sought to normalize sex consumption by using the party planning technique pioneered by Tupperware in the 1950s (Smith 2007), with their website claiming 'There are over 2,500 parties held each week by over 5,000 dedicated ambassadors across the UK' (cited in Maginn and Steinmitz 2015: 30).

In the words of *Ann Summers'* CEO, Jacqueline Gold, the aim of the chain has been to make a visit to the store 'part of a regular shopping trip', and to that end the chain has sought high-profile locations on the High Street and even in shopping malls (there's one at Bluewater, for example, only a couple of units down from the *Build-a-Bear* workshop). The chain has been able to do this partly by trading on its feminized identity, but also by describing itself as a 'passion and fashion' shop, and not a sex shop. In legal terms, this distinction is validated by the fact it does not stock the R18 pornographic DVDs that can only be sold with a local authority sex shop licence; in design terms, the majority of floor space is devoted to lingerie, with sex toys, lubricants and bondage gear located more discretely at the back of the store. These types of tactics have ensured corporate property owners have been happy to rent premises to *Ann Summers* in prominent retail locations. And while a recent rebrand designed to make the store more appealing to the 18–35 demographic has resulted in the gradual replacement of the pink façade by a new, racier 'black store', seemingly, there's very few complaints received about the way that these stores project 'sexiness' onto the High Street. This said, sometimes even *Ann Summers* oversteps the mark: a *50 Shades of Grey*-inspired 'Bring the Film To Life' poster featuring a woman with a peep-hole bra was removed from the windows of several shops in 2015 after Mediawatch concluded 'We are used to seeing the windows of *Ann Summers* featuring lingerie but this image, featuring a bare-breasted (except for nipple tassels) model goes too far and is inappropriate for display in places which are likely to have numbers of children present'.

So, despite the claim that commercial sex constitutes the 'lowest' of all cultural products (see Papayanis 2000), *Ann Summers* has seemingly prospered on the High Street because it has challenged the stereotype of 'the fantasy pornography consumer who is a walking projection of upper-class fears about lower class men: brutish, animal-like and sexually vora-cious' (Kipnis 1996: 174). Far from being viewed as out of place on the High Street, *Ann Summers* and other erotic boutiques are imbued with symbolic capital that ensures they are deemed to be part of a thriving, and even gentrified, retail offer. Here, the collision of consumer medi-ated subjectivities and publicly visible sexualities is complex, but the idea that women are now able to choose how they present their own bodies as objects of desire seems crucial in cementing the idea that sex retailing on the High Street is acceptable, so long as it's aimed at women. As Evans et al. (2010: 115) argue, 'the sexualisation of contemporary British cul-ture has in part been enabled by a neo-liberal rhetoric of agency, choice and self-determination, which within sexuality discourses have produced an "up for it" femininity, a sexually savvy and active woman who can participate appropriately in consumer practices in the production of her choice biography'. Even though the role model is provided by the kinky but passive heterosexuality of *50 Shades of Grey*, circuits of female con-sumption are set in motion, which reproduce sexuality as a valued com-modity (Dymock 2013).

While it has not 'poshed up' its products in quite the same way that *Coco de Mer* or *Agent Provocateur* have (Carter 2014), *Anne Summers* is then a gentrified sex shop, having taken sex consumption to the middle classes by focusing on sex-positive images of women that bestow value and status on those who spend money on sexy products. In contrast, the licensed sex shop—no matter how much it tries to depict itself as 'couple-oriented'—remains subject to a licensing regime that is responsive to complaints from those who continue to regard pornography as a lower-class commodity existing solely for the gratification of men. Indeed, Melissa Tyler (2011) argues that it's the existence of this masculinized, seedy 'Other' in the sex-retailing sector that allows feminization and gentrification to work hand in hand. But the *Ann Summers* ethos can be questioned given that it does not fundamentally disrupt traditional images of feminine desirability, and valorizes white, middle-class heterosexual norms. Moreover, it does little to tackle the objectification of women's sexuality within a 'pornified' culture, with its stores playing a role in mainstreaming ideas that women are sexually available. Indeed, within a city where an excess of sexualized images is sometimes accused of dominating public space (Kalms 2014), the window displays of *Ann Summers* are often indistinguishable from the digital media, billboards and posters that commodify women's sexuality using provocative and sometimes pseudo-pornographic imagery. While such traditions of using the female form to promote consumption are not new, the explicit nature of many contemporary images raises particular concerns about the visibility of sex on our High Streets:

> Of course the body as a site for economic exchange is neither new nor surprising—nor is the ever-shifting territory of what constitutes 'public'. What has changed for both sexuality and publicness is the relationship between urban form and the contemporary media. Furthermore, the sexualised events of urban life—once contained and controlled in interior spaces—are now moving into and onto the public realm. This is the hyper-sexual condition. (Kalms 2014: 381)

The idea that ever-present images of sexualized bodies on billboards, signage and advertising hoardings render the city a sexual marketplace where bodies are constantly on display, and all is for sale has been a prominent theme in contemporary feminist scholarship on the city (Rosewarne 2009). For some, this fundamentally changes the nature of women's engagement with the city centre, and risks making the High Street into a 'no go' zone for unaccompanied women. So while sex shops aimed at women appear to have been accepted, it's not clear as to whether they help to alter the fundamentally gendered nature of the public sphere. However, this is an argument that has been much more pronounced in relation to one of the most controversial venues on the contemporary British High Street: the lap dance or striptease club.

Lap Dance Clubs: Resisting the 'Hypersexualization' of Cities

The arrival of the 'US style' lap dance club in Britain in the late 1990s appeared to symbolize something fairly significant in terms of the 'mainstreaming' of commercial sexuality. For sure, striptease dancing had long been available in British cities for those who sought it out, but was a largely clandestine affair, occurring principally in 'working men's' pubs and clubs. But the opening of corporate 'gentleman's clubs' like *Spearmint Rhino* and *For Your Eyes Only* on the High Street seemed to suggest that striptease was both a legitimate and highly profitable form of entertainment. The branding of striptease as 'adult entertainment' for the discerning 'gentleman' was significant, as it sought to replace images of cheap, sordid entertainment with something altogether more stylish. Gentleman's clubs were manifestly not venues that encouraged high-volume alcohol consumption through cheap drinks promotions. Instead, these venues promoted an image of urbane sophistication, envisioning an audience prepared to pay a premium to drink champagne while it was indulged with highly sexualized entertainment in private booths. Fitting into certain ideas about the importance of catering to business travellers and corporate clients, striptease flourished in new purpose-built clubs, being seen as 'a stylish, up-market and respectable form of entertainment' which also conformed with discourses concerning the desirability of cultivating a 'continental' 24-hour city (Chatterton and Hollands 2003: 158–160). It was little wonder many struggling pubs decided to rebrand themselves as lap dance venues in the hope of attracting a more affluent clientele (or at least one prepared to spend more on drinks). While no-one seems quite sure how many dedicated clubs there were, a figure of around 350 in 2004 seems a reasonable estimate, meaning every major town and city in Britain possessed at least one club at that time.

However, the backlash against lap dancing clubs was not long in coming, and when it did, it was considerable. While opposition was fairly muted when the first clubs appeared in the West End of London, the fact that almost every British High Street possessed a lap dance club by the early 2000s meant the debate became a national one, mediated by a national press arguing this 'US-led invasion' had resulted in an 'epidemic of sleaze on the High Street' with 'tawdry lap dance clubs springing up all over Britain' (Rawstorne 2008: np). Sexual entertainment was seemingly fair enough in central London, but when clubs opened in 'middle class market towns like Stourbridge', or 50 yards from a church in Oxford, in 'genteel' Leamington Spa or even in 'solid Guardian reader territory' like Crouch End in North London, the headlines were predictable. In each case, proposed clubs were opposed by a mix of anxious residents, enraged councillors and concerned religious leaders (see Hubbard 2009). Such protests drew sustenance from an emergent national campaign spearheaded by *Object*, a feminist group opposing the objectification of women. Accusing sexual entertainment of coarsening the city, creating no-go zones for women, and of normalizing retrogressive, male attitudes towards women, *Object's* key contention was that such venues were subject to insufficient state regulation, noting it was possible to put on lap dance in any licensed premises so long as there were no valid objections received from those living within 100 metres (Hadfield and Measham 2009: 6). For *Object*, this treated lap dance clubs the same as a pub, club or coffee shop, something they found bewildering given the type of entertainment on offer:

> Lap dancing clubs are venues where customers pay female performers to visually sexually stimulate them by pole dancing, table dancing or gyrating on their lap whilst removing most or all of their clothing to expose genitals and excretory organs. It's clear that as part of the commercial sex industry they have more in common with peep shows and sex cinemas than with *Pizza Express* or *Odeon* cinemas. (Object 2008: 8)

In light of such discourses of opposition, the government passed the *Policing and Crime Act 2009* allowing for a more rigorous licensing of such venues, empowering local authorities to refuse licences for such venues in areas regarded as inappropriate by adding clauses to the 1982 Act that had been introduced to control sex shops. The subsequent licensing of such clubs as Sexual Entertainment Venues (SEVs), and the continuing 'backlash' against them, has meant their numbers have subsided from around 350 in 2004 to fewer than 180 dedicated clubs at the end of 2015. At least 50 clubs have seen licence applications or renewals refused by local authority committees, mainly on grounds of inappropriate locality and seldom with any police objection or evidence of criminality or nuisance in the vicinity. These closures have sometimes had devastating consequences for venue owners and employees alike (see Sanders and Hardy 2012 on precarity in the lap dance industry). Nonetheless, each closure is heralded as a success in terms of improving community safety, and making women in particular feel more comfortable in an evening economy 'blighted' by such premises.

In the face of the national and local campaigns orchestrated against lap dancing, asking whether the enforced closure of clubs has actually been detrimental to the creation of vibrant and vital High Streets appears somewhat churlish. Indeed, it's a question few besides the managers and owners of lap dance clubs have posed. But one article commenting on the situation in Leeds dares to raise this very question, noting that there had been a push to close down a number of the city's clubs in advance of the arrival of the prestigious *Tour De France* in 2014:

> There were those who were seemingly racing against time to rid the city centre of some of its lap-dancing bars before the eyes of the world started to turn to Leeds. They were adamant that having these establishments in such prominent, city centre locations (including right on the start line of the aforementioned cycle race) was not in keeping with the modern, cosmopolitan city we wanted everyone to remember us as when the big event had come and gone. On the other were those who insisted such bars should stay open, that they weren't doing any harm and that a vocal minority shouldn't be clamouring to run local, long-established businesses out of town. Whatever side you're on, the legacy of that decision has been the fact

that ever since then, we've been left with some huge vacant sites in some very prominent places across the city … it's almost been a year since the *Tour de France*—and two years since some of the venues had to close—and yet these bars are still lying there empty. (Time for Some Naked Ambition over Former Leeds lap dancing venues? *Yorkshire Evening Post*, 19 April 2015)

It's worth noting here that the three Leeds lap dance clubs which lost their licence—*Deep Blue, Wildcats* and *Red Leopard*—did so despite 1649 survey responses to a Leeds City Council survey revealing only 39% objected to striptease clubs in the city centre (as against 49% claiming these locations were suitable). Despite this seemingly ambivalent set of results, the Council Licensing Sub-committee, encouraged by local MPs who argued that the number of premises needed to be significantly reduced, especially near 'prominent' venues such as the City Art Gallery, Town Hall and War Memorial, refused licences 'due to the number of buildings with sensitive uses nearby to the location of the premises'.

The implication of this—as well as similar refusals elsewhere (Hubbard 2015)—is that the desire to drive lap dance clubs off the High Street appears to reflect anxiety about place image rather than any evidence of criminality in or around such clubs. Indeed, in a national study of local residents' attitudes towards venues in their local town or city centre (n = 941), we found that sexual entertainment venues were not regarded as a significant source of nuisance or anxiety by the majority of residents. Overall, lap dance clubs were regarded significantly less likely to create anti-social behaviour, noise or littering than other pubs or clubs, although 58% agreed that their presence lowered the reputation of their town or city (see Hubbard and Colosi 2015). But these results varied according to age, class and gender. Older home-owners were more opposed to lap dance clubs than younger groups, with two-thirds of 18–24 year olds stating the number of striptease clubs was 'about right', contrasting with the two-thirds of over 40s arguing there were 'too many'. One in three of our respondents also claimed to feel reasonably or very unsafe walking at night in cities with lap dance clubs. This group was significantly more likely to say there were too many striptease clubs in their town than those who felt safe, and more likely than any other group to say they would avoid walking past a lap dance club at night. Perhaps unsurprisingly, women were significantly over-represented in this group, suggesting the presence of sexual entertainment in the night-time city may have gendered effects. It is something we explored further in a series of guided nighttime walks in four towns with lap dance clubs. These mixed-gender walks confirmed women were more likely to note, and comment on, the presence of striptease clubs in their local towns than men. Yet here, it appeared that unease about striptease clubs was more related to questions of class, morality and disgust than fear, with these clubs' contribution to anti-social and rowdy behaviour deemed lesser than that associated with many other local venues such as the clubs, pubs and takeaways which seemed to enjoy particular notoriety amongst our participants as spaces of drunken and disorderly behaviour.

This suggests that objections to lap dance clubs are related to what they appear to stand for as much as what happens in and around them. Indeed, the vast majority of those who object to lap dance clubs seem only dimly aware of what happens in clubs, but this does not prevent them from articulating a general discourse of opposition that portrays lap dance clubs as, in the words of one respondent, 'sleazy, objectionable and offensive':

> Well I have to say I hate the thought of having one here. I've never heard any rowdy behaviour or anything. But I don't like the thought of lap dancing, I think that it's just tacky. (Respondent on guided walk, Maidstone, Female, 50s)

Such narratives emphasizing the immorality of lap dancing suggest that the presence of a club precipitates a process of local decline, something echoed in the type of objections received by local authorities; such as:

> The tone of the neighbourhood will be lowered, residents will think twice before leaving their property in the evening. There will be reduction in property value—people will not want to live near such and undesirable business. (Letter in opposition to relicensing of *Spearmint Rhino*, appendix 14, 24 May 2012, Camden Licensing Committee)

Or:

> This area has historically suffered from a stigmatized image and efforts have
> been made to regenerate the area to benefit businesses and residents alike.
> The presence of a sex industry premises confounds this image and under-
> mines such efforts. (Letter in opposition to licensing of *Shades*, Leamington
> Spa, 19 July 2012, Warwick District Council Licensing Subcommittee).

Hence, although there are occasional concerns aired about the impact of
clubs on local crime rates, far more numerous are discourses describing
these venues as potentially degrading urban centres: the 58% believing
that the presence of a club decreases the reputation of a town/city was
double the proportion suggesting it reduces safety on the street.

Here, anxieties about clubs, where expressed, appear particularly
related to concerns about the debasement of civic life, and particularly
the overt representation of sexuality through club signage, names and flyers (Fig. 6.2). Indeed, we found a dominant feeling among respondents
that venues should be 'low key' and inconspicuous; those with children
feared having to explain to them the nature of the entertainment which
takes place inside if asked. One of our respondents relayed her experience:

> The one on [*this road*], I can remember my son asking 'what's that then?',
> having a conversation with my husband and I was just thinking how do
> you explain that to a six year old who's completely innocent? I don't know,
> since I've had children it bothers me but I think before I wouldn't have
> given it much thought. (Respondent on guided walk, Newcastle, Female,
> 40s)

A key theme that emerged from our roving interviews was an anxiety
about the way that lap dance clubs advertised their presence, shifting
what Anne Cronin (2006) terms the 'metabolism of the city' by sexual-
izing particular streets at particular times. It has been argued elsewhere
that sexualized advertisements make women feel uneasy on a number of
levels, with the display of pseudo-pornographic pictures and women in a
state of semi-nudity constituting a form of sexual harassment (Rosewarne
2009), something around which guidelines have developed (such as
those developed by the Advertising Standards Authority in the UK). It
was noted by several of our respondents that overtly sexist images and

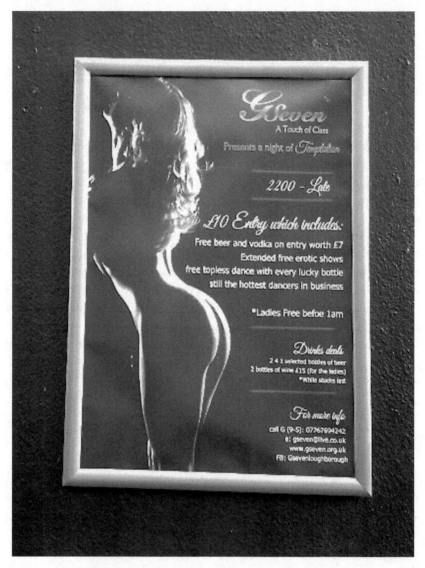

Fig. 6.2 A touch of class? Poster outside now-defunct Gentleman's Club G7, Loughborough 2013 (photo: author)

representations were routinely embedded in urban space through club's flyers, advertising boards and signage. While local authorities demand that advertising is discrete and non-explicit, the names of clubs (e.g. *Beavers*, Watford, *Pussy Galore*, Newcastle-upon-Tyne, *Bottoms Up!*, Edinburgh) are sometimes far from subtle, with ever-present images of sexualized white, blonde, slim, female bodies on premises' façades being used to seduce the (assumed male, heterosexual) viewer:

> The advertising material consists of a display board with colourful writing advertising exotic dancers with the image of a silhouette of a pole dancer. This type of material is highly visible to any tourist or visitor … the promotion of these activities makes the High Street seem seedy and uninviting. (Representation against a venue in Rochester, Medway Council licensing committee, 23 October 2011)

Under the terms of the new licensing regime for lap dance clubs, local authorities are able to demand no part of the interior of a club is visible from the outside, concealing the nature of the entertainment from passers-by (as per the traditional sex shop). The idea that the external appearance of a club is all important was played up by several participants in our go-along interviews, including one who suggested a club contributed to 'a sleazy atmosphere with its blacked out windows' and another which argued 'it just looks sinister'. This suggests that lap dance clubs can effectively sexualize the High Street via aesthetics of concealment and seduction. In this sense, class, immorality and deviance were connected via the materialization of lap dance clubs in the landscape, leading to anxious and defensive middle-class reactions based on disgust and exclusion (see Hubbard and Colosi 2015).

This kind of assessment underlines Sara Ahmed's argument that disgust reactions do not simply result from an encounter with a 'primary object of disgust' (such as the naked body) but contact with the other signs and objects that stand in for it. As she argues:

> The way in which disgust is generated by 'contact' between objects is what makes the attribution of disgust dependent on a certain history, rather than being a necessary consequence of the nature of things. It is not that an

object we might encounter is inherently disgusting; rather, an object becomes disgusting through its contact with other objects that have already, as it were, been designated as disgusting before the encounter has taken place. It is the dependency of disgust on contact or proximity that may explain its awkward temporality, the way it both lags behind the objects from which it recoils and generates the object in the moment of recoiling. (Ahmed 2013: 87)

Here, disgust is described as an emotion shaped by contact with an object that is associated with dirt, rather than being caused by the dirt of the object per se, affective experience being 'a cumulative, and therefore historical, process of interaction between human beings and place' (Kobayashi et al. 2011: 873). This geographically informed perspective on disgust suggests the interpretation of middle-class standards of behaviour and comportment needs to be understood relationally, with the transgression of 'civilized' standards of behaviour judged contextually in the context of particular representations and images, which in themselves are not necessarily disgusting.

The implication here is that the naked body itself is not always interpreted as disgusting—far from it—but that the mimetic representation of the female body as an overt (and purchasable) sex symbol is something capable of provoking languages of disgust. As reflected in media coverage at the national level, as much as in local discourses of opposition, lap dance clubs are accused of undermining respectable femininity by presenting the female body as a sex object to be consumed by a male viewer. So, while some forms of striptease (e.g. burlesque) are frequently described in playful terms as a cultured celebration of feminine desire or sexuality; lap dance is frequently regarded to be seen as lacking value because of the assumed gendered dynamic of women being sexually objectified by a male clientele. Despite venues describing themselves as 'gentleman's clubs', a common trope has been the identification of this clientele as a working-class 'Other', unable to appreciate the performance of striptease artistes except in a base, carnal manner.

Though participants in our study were drawn from a variety of class positions and backgrounds, they hence strove to locate themselves within middle-class frames of conduct by suggesting that the description of some lap dance venues as 'gentleman's clubs' was a misnomer:

No gentlemen would frequent a bar like this. I think if he was to say: 'no I'm not going to frequent such things that are degrading'—I would maybe think of him more of a gentleman. (Respondent on Guided Walk, Newcastle, Female, 30s)

This type of moral judgment labels the clients of lap dance establishments as failing to exercise civilized, middle-class taste, with the (assumed male) clients described in pejorative terms. This chimes with the allegations made in letters opposing the licensing of sexual entertainment venues, where the behaviour of clients is often described in similar terms:

Our street serves as the car park for the groups of often drunk, loud and obscene punters who roll up, clearly seeing a visit to a lap-dancing club as the end of a glorious night's drinking. These men travel in packs, and engage in displays of bravado, frequently swearing, urinating in gardens and egging each other on … Nobody in our neighbourhood can take a walk without risking encounters with the clients. (Letter of opposition against a venue, London Borough of Richmond on Thames licensing subcommittee, 29 July 2010)

The deployment of animalistic metaphors (i.e. travelling in packs) hints at the projection of non-human traits onto stigmatized groups (Rozin and Fallon 1987; Sibley 1995), and constructs a moral hierarchy in which those who purchase sexual entertainment are constructed as 'as dehumanized, dirty and animalistic' (Campbell and Storr 2001: 98). Sarah Kingston (2013: 17) argues there's often little difference in the language used to describe those who buy sex and those who consume sexual entertainment: both are portrayed as a 'predator who needs to be guarded against, external to the community of "normal" men—an outsider who is untrustworthy and "dangerous"'. As one of the participants in our guided walks commented 'in the club the local women are yours for the taking if you want and then they [men] have a drink, and this then progresses onto the streets, and when they're in their packs and if you happen to be there … who knows what' (respondent on guided walk, Newcastle, Female, 30s).

There's some degree of conflation here between the clientele of the lap dance club and the stereotyped 'lager louts' commonly depicted as 'literally spilling out of one drinking den into the next one and, all the while, representing the potential for disorder and the transgression of propriety' (Thurnell-Read 2013: np). Multiple representations against lap dance clubs hence allude to possibility that 'patrons who are generally intoxicated and arguably in a state of sexual excitement' might harass local women, noting that venues often target 'stag parties which are renowned for their negative impact in relation to crime and disorder' (representations 51, 52, and 52a, Bristol City Council licensing committee 13 October 2011). For instance, one of our participants during a guided walk expressed her anxiety about the effect of venues on men, suggesting they put female members of the public at risk as '… it's just feeding men frenzy, and then they go out on the street and we [*women*] get all the shit' (respondent on guided walk, Lincoln, Female, 40s). However, the same respondent stressed she had not actually witnessed or personally experienced any threatening behaviour while in close proximity to a lap dance club, suggesting that her fears were based on the stigmatizing discourses that surround this maligned industry. Indeed, allegations of serious sexual assaults perpetrated by clients against women appear extremely rare, with the most frequent accusations being that clubs attract 'unsavoury' male visitors who made the areas around clubs feel unsafe for female passers-by (see Hubbard and Colosi 2015). While most academic studies of the lap dance industry are from the USA, the vast majority show little or no relationship between the presence of clubs and criminality—and where crimes are more pronounced, it appears the most 'at risk' group are those men attending clubs, who are prone to mugging and personal attack on the basis that they are often carrying large amounts of cash and might be reticent to report a crime that happened outside or near a strip club (see Seaman and Linz 2014).

Sanitizing the High Street?

Arguably, there's a big difference between shops selling 'sex products' on the High Street and venues where bodies are sexually consumed. Nonetheless, the rhetoric surrounding the rise of lap dance clubs on British High Streets mirrors that which circulated around the emergence of 'traditional' sex shop in earlier decades. Both spaces have been depicted as sordid, dirty, even dangerous, and their clientele known through myths of deviance. Discourses of opposition to both sex shops and lap dance clubs project negative values onto the 'disrespectable' working class assumed to be their main customers. This public condemnation of sexual consumption undoubtedly plays an important role in the reproduction of dominant notions of civility, morality and gendered respectability, the expression of disgust towards it being one means used by middle-class subjects to claim respectability. Distinction is then expressed through a language of disgust, with this being used to demonstrate that the Self is cultured and civilized. As such, it appears impossible to reproduce anything other than a classed discourse about sexual consumption—even if this is sometimes manifest in a language which appears more about maintaining community standards rather than condemning working-class identities outright (see also Skeggs 1997, on dis-identification).

Given this, it's hardly surprising that sex establishments are among the most vilified premises on our High Streets, with a Local Government Association (2012) survey suggesting that clusters of strip clubs and sex shops were more likely than any other retail premises to have a negative effect on the vibrancy of a local shopping centre. Those who consider the consumption of sexual entertainment as harmless, good fun, or a viable form of employment for women in recessionary times, appear badly out of step with public opinion. It appears that to publicly admit to enjoying, or even tolerating, sexual entertainment is to admit a lack of taste, identifying one as devoid of value, and immoral. And while we apparently live in 'pornified' times, sex-related commerce remains to be regarded with suspicion, associated with an industry that remains 'dirty work' (Tyler 2011). The opposition expressed to sex establishments can hence be interpreted as part of an attempt to police the boundaries of middle-class respectability, 'othering' the producers and consumers of commercial sex through 'speech acts' that identify them as an affront to public decency. As we have seen, the language used to describe the male clientele of lap dance clubs echoes wider concerns about working-class masculinities on the night-time High Street (Thurnell-Read 2013), while the disgust registered about women selling sexualized performances repeats long-standing stereotypes of working-class women as wanton, immoral and exploited.

In the case of both sex shops and lap dance clubs, the state has responded to these popular fears and disgusts by introducing regulations designed to give local authorities more power to remove these premises from given localities. In both instances, the forms of regulation enacted by the state allow it to claim that it's uninterested in questions of private sexual morality, and is not interfering in the rights of adults to consume sexual materials. The legislation introduced—at great expense to the local authorities charged with enforcing the new sex establishment licensing regime—does not criminalize the consumption of commercial sex, but merely stipulates that it cannot occur in 'inappropriate localities'. The fact that few British local authorities have made any effort to identify areas where sex shops or lap dance clubs might actually be acceptable underlines that it's down to individual operators to demonstrate that their premises might actually not cause major offence. In general terms, this adversarial process has favoured the more corporate, 'well-managed' sex establishments that can afford good licensing lawyers capable of constructing an argument that their business might actually be good for the local economy. The larger lap dance chains—*Spearmint Rhino and For Your Eyes Only*—continue to prosper, while the less well-funded, smaller operators have been pushed away from prime High Street locations even in a time of recession when it's by no means clear what alternative businesses might replace them. 'Queer' businesses, including gay burlesque nights, clubs featuring dark rooms, and gay saunas, appear particularly vulnerable here, with one of London's main areas of gay nightlife (Vauxhall) appearing threatened by the combination of the new licensing regime and rising rents.

While it's tempting to describe this de facto gentrification of sex businesses as a planned regulatory outcome, it's perhaps best viewed as the messy, cumulative outcome of local decision-making processes biased towards the moral and aesthetic values of the middle class, and particularly middle-aged property owners and developers (Valverde 2012). But in this context, what are we to make of the presence of female-oriented sex shops on gentrified, commercially successful High Streets? Why have these stores evaded regulation even though much of their stock is manifestly and unambiguously related to sexual pleasures? Perhaps it's because, in High Streets where 'unhealthy' businesses seemingly abound (e.g. shops offering cheap alcohol, fast food, legal highs), shops like *Ann*

Summers appear surprisingly wholesome, celebrating the idea that women can enjoy a fulfilling and healthy sex life. Myths of autonomy and emancipation abound, bequeathing the female consumer of sex products with a form of respectability long denied to male consumers. So even though urban policy sometimes appears resolutely 'anti-sexual', there's clearly still a place for sex on the High Street, so long as it's packaged appropriately, and does not disturb middle-class norms of respectability. Even Mary Portas has endorsed her own range of Kinky Knickers.

References

Ahmed, S. (2013). *The cultural politics of emotion*. London: Routledge.

Astrup, J. (2013). Shock as sex shop opens near school uniform store. *Daily Echo*, 17 May http://www.dailyecho.co.uk/news/10428401. Shock_as_sex_shop_opens_near_school_uniform_store/

Campbell, R., & Storr, M. (2001). Challenging the kerb-crawler rehabilitation programme. *Feminist Review, 67*(1), 94–108.

Carter, F. (2014). Magic toyshops. In A. Moran & S. O'Brien (Eds.), *Love objects*. London: Bloomsbury.

Chatterton, P., & Hollands, R. (2003). *Urban nightscapes: Youth cultures, pleasure spaces and corporate power*. London: Routledge.

Coulmont, B., & Hubbard, P. (2010). Consuming sex: Socio-legal shifts in the space and place of sex shops. *Journal of Law and Society, 37*(1), 189–209.

Cronin, A. M. (2006). Advertising and the metabolism of the city: Urban space, commodity rhythms. *Environment and Planning D: Society and Space, 24*(4), 615–632.

Dymock, A. (2013). Flogging sexual transgression: Interrogating the costs of the 'fifty shades effect'. *Sexualities, 16*(8), 880–895.

Edwards, M. L. (2010). Gender, social disorganization theory, and the locations of sexually oriented businesses. *Deviant Behavior, 31*(2), 135–158.

Evans, A., Riley, S., & Shankar, A. (2010). Postfeminist heterotopias negotiating 'safe' and 'seedy' in the British sex shop space. *European Journal of Women's Studies, 17*(3), 211–229.

Foucault, M. (1991). Governmentality. In G. Burchell, C. Gordon, & P. Miller (Eds.), *The Foucault effect: Studies in governmentality*. Chicago, IL: University of Chicago Press.

Hadfield, P., & Measham, F. (2009). Shaping the night: How licensing, social divisions and informal social controls mould the form and content of nightlife. *Crime Prevention & Community Safety, 11*(3), 219–234.

Hubbard, P. (2009). Opposing striptopia: The embattled spaces of adult entertainment. *Sexualities, 12*(6), 721–745.

Hubbard, P. (2013). Carnage! Coming to a town near you? Nightlife, uncivilised behaviour and the carnivalesque body. *Leisure Studies, 32*(3), 265–282.

Hubbard, P. (2015). Law, sex and the city: Regulating sexual entertainment venues in England and Wales. *International Journal of Law in the Built Environment, 7*(1), 5–20.

Hubbard, P., & Colosi, R. (2015). Respectability, morality and disgust in the night-time economy: Exploring reactions to 'lap dance' clubs in England and Wales. *The Sociological Review, 63*(4), 782–800.

Hunter, I., Saunders, D., & Williamson, D. (1993). *On pornography: Literature, sexuality, and obscenity law*. Basingstoke: Macmillan.

Kalms, N. (2014). Provocations of the hypersexualized city. *Architecture and Culture, 2*(3), 379–402.

Kingston, S. (2013). *Prostitution in the community*. London: Routledge.

Kipnis, L. (1996). *Bound and gagged*. New York: Grove Press.

Kobayashi, A., Preston, V., & Murnaghan, A. (2011). Place, affect, and transnationalism through the voices of Hong Kong immigrants to Canada. *Social and Cultural Geography, 12*(4), 871–888.

Kristeva, J. (1982). *Powers of horror*. New York: Columbia University Press.

Laing, M. (2012). Regulating adult work in Canada: The role of criminal and municipal code. In P. Johnson & D. Dalton (Eds.), *Policing sex*. London: Routledge.

Legg, S. (2005). Foucault's population geographies: Classifications, biopolitics and governmental spaces. *Population, Space and Place, 11*(3), 137–156.

Local Government Association (2012) LGA Survey—Strip clubs and bookies are hitting economic growth. LGA media release, 14 April 2012, http://www.local.gov.uk/media-centre/-/journal_content/56/10180/3376601/NEWS

Maginn, P., & Steinmetz, C. (2015). Spatial and regulatory contours of the sex industry. In P. Maginn & C. Steinmetz (Eds.), *(Sub)urban sexscape: Geographies and regulation of the sex industry* (pp. 1–16). London: Routledge.

Malina, D., & Schmidt, R. A. (1997). It's business doing pleasure with you: Sh! A women's sex shop case. *Marketing Intelligence & Planning, 15*(7), 352–360.

Manchester, C. (1990). Refusing the renewal of sex establishment licences. *The Modern Law Review, 53*(2), 248–255.

Martin, A. (2013). Fifty shades of sex shop: Sexual fantasy for sale. *Sexualities, 16*(8), 980–984.

Object. (2008). *Stripping the illusion.* London: Object.

Papayanis, M. A. (2000). Sex and the revanchist city: Zoning out pornography in New York. *Environment and Planning D, 18*(3), 341–354.

Peter Brett Associates (2013). Poole and Purbeck Town Centres retail and leisure study. Bristol, Peter Brett on behalf of Poole and Purbeck Councils.

Rawstorne, T. (2008). Tawdry lap dancing clubs are springing up all over Britain. Who is to blame for this epidemic of sleaze on the High Street? The Mail on Sunday, 21 June, http://www.dailymail.co.uk/news/article-1028078/Tawdry-lap-dancing-clubs-springing-Britain–whos-blame-epidemic-sleaze-High-Street.html

Rosewarne, L. (2009). *Sex in public: Women, outdoor advertising, and public policy.* Newcastle: Cambridge Scholars Publishing.

Rozin, P., & Fallon, A. E. (1987). A perspective on disgust. *Psychological Review, 94*(1), 23.

Sanders, T., & Hardy, K. (2012). Devalued, deskilled and diversified: Explaining the proliferation of the strip industry in the UK. *British Journal of Sociology, 63*(3), S13–S32.

Seaman, C., & Linz, D. (2014). Are adult businesses crime hotspots? Comparing adult businesses to other locations in three cities. *Journal of Criminology.* Retrieved from http://www.hindawi.com/journals/jcrim/2014/783461/

Shildrick, M. (1997). *Leaky bodies and boundaries: Feminism, postmodernism and (bio)ethics.* London: Routlege.

Sibley, D. (1995). *Geographies of exclusion: Society and difference in the west.* London: Routledge.

Skeggs, B. (1997). *Formations of class & gender: Becoming respectable.* London: Sage.

Smith, C. (2007). *One for the girls!: The pleasures and practices of reading women's porn.* London: Intellect Books.

Thurnell-Read, T. (2013). 'Yobs' and 'Snobs': Embodying drink and the problematic male drinking body. *Sociological Research Online, 18*(2), 3.

Tyler, M. (2011). Tainted love: From dirty work to abject labour in Soho's sex shops. *Human Relations, 64*(11), 1477–1500.

Tyler, M. (2012). 'Glamour girls, macho men and everything in between': Un/doing gender and dirty work in Soho's sex shops. In R. Simpson, N. Slutskaya, P. Lewis, & H. Höpfl (Eds.), *Dirty work: Concepts and identities.* Palgrave Macmillan: Basingstoke.

Valverde, M. (2012). *Everyday law on the street: City governance in an age of diversity*. Toronto: University of Chicago Press.

Van der Meulen, E., & Valverde, M. (2013). Beyond the criminal code: Municipal licensing and zoning bylaws. In E. Van Der Meulen, E. Duirisin, & V. Love (Eds.), *Selling sex: Experience, advocacy, and research on sex work in Canada*. Vancouver: UBC Press.

7

Place Your Bets

In the early 2000s, New Labour politicians presented gambling as a possible solution to the economic and social problems being faced by struggling communities. The Department of Culture, Media and Sport (2002) went so far as to identify gambling as 'a safe bet' for economic and job creation, arguing for liberalization of what were still paternalistic and patchwork regulations essentially aimed at 'protecting' gamblers. Crucially, this shifted the discussion about gambling from one about criminality and vice to one in which the gambling industry was seen as thoroughly capable of contributing in a meaningful way to the leisure economy. The *Gambling Act 2005* hence dethroned magistrates—long responsible for issuing gaming licenses—with local authorities taking over the licensing of bingo halls, betting shops and casinos (Bedford 2011). This was especially significant given talk of Las Vegas style 'regional casinos' had encouraged the government to hold a competition to authorize 16 regional casinos (of up to 1000 square metres) alongside one national super-casino of up to 5000 square metres (including 1250 gaming machines). Many towns and cities began to jockey for the award of the super-casino licence, with Manchester given permission to develop this in 2007, much to the surprise of frontrunner Blackpool, which had

© The Editor(s) (if applicable) and The Author(s) 2017   **147**
P. Hubbard, *The Battle for the High Street*,
DOI 10.1057/978-1-137-52153-8_7

argued the award would provide a timely stimulus to its declining tourism and entertainment sector.

But at the same moment that the gambling industry and national politicians enthused about the possibilities of using gambling as a means of urban regeneration, counter views emerged, effectively killing the idea that casinos could rejuvenate and enliven local economic development. As Graham Brooks details (2012), this involved a campaign orchestrated by *The Daily Mail* to 'kill the bill'—a campaign which presented gambling as immoral and sinful, a precursor to criminality rather than an engine of economic growth. No wonder the award of a super-casino licence to Manchester was ultimately defeated in the House of Lords, with the enthusiasm for gambling de-regulation tempered by a realization there was still a significant lobby regarding it as a disease. The marginalized, unemployed and 'socially vulnerable' were represented as unable to make rational choices, with gambling referred to as a temptation which the 'poor' were unable to resist. The government became portrayed as a 'peddler' of addiction, with the individual and collective 'poor' potential victims of gambling's irresistible attraction (Brooks 2012: 745).

Yet, while much of the discussion about the rights and wrongs of gambling de-regulation has centred on casinos—which number around 140 in the UK—these sites are relatively insignificant in job creation terms compared to licensed bingo halls (around 640) and betting shops (well over 8000). In contrast to casinos, bingo halls have rarely been figured as risky sites: while casinos have been depicted as turning even the most sensible individual into a problem gambler as soon as they cross the threshold, bingo remains depicted as harmless fun, and not 'real gambling' (Bedford 2011: 377). Betting shops, however, remain a different matter, and in the last decade much of the anxiety about gambling has shifted from debates concerning the potential for Las Vegas tourist type super-casinos to transform local economies to the existence of bookmakers on the High Street. Far from being seen as a virtuous presence, betting shops have become depicted as a noxious presence on the High Street, another of the 'toxic' businesses tainting local shopping streets (Townshend 2016) by peddling a product linked with misery and exploitation.

Betting Shops as a Noxious Business

Croydon has long been one of London's least loved suburbs. In the 1960s it underwent massive redevelopment, bequeathing it with a modernist town centre that remains excitingly futurist or tremendously boring, depending on your perspective. And while it's the largest London borough by population, with more commuters journeying in and out of East Croydon station every day than Edinburgh Waverley or Liverpool Lime Street, its town centre still has more vacant properties and lower footfall than the national average (GLA 2014). Like many other towns, the retail core, built around a shopping centre (*The Whitgift*, first opened in 1970), is not faring too badly (around 15% vacant in 2012) but the fringe areas of London Road and the 'Old Town' have vacancy rates of more than one in five units empty. The latter area became a 'Portas Pilot' in 2012, part of the first tranche of projects funded by the DCLG, and set about revitalizing the area's street market and encouraging independent traders. London Road, on the other hand, was badly affected by looting and fire-damage in the 'English riots' of 2011, prompting grant support for small businesses in the hope of rebuilding confidence in this area. The Mayor of London's office and Croydon Council provided Business Rate Relief and 90% funding for shop façade 'smartening' in an effort to 'build on the area's ethnic shopping offer, address the physical issues along the London Road … change perceptions of the area and attract new people' (GLA 2012).

In this light, the planned takeover of a vacant *Chicken Cottage* store on London Road by national bookmakers' chain *Paddy Power* might have been greeted positively by the local community, given that it promised new jobs and a new business in an area struggling in the wake of the retail recession. Yet the application for a betting licence for the premises (required under the terms of the *Gambling Act 2005*) was made in the face of 48 objections, including several from local councillors, organizations working with the local Tamil population, local traders and members of West Croydon Community Forum, with a spokesperson for the latter arguing:

> West Croydon is becoming awash with betting offices, pawnshops and moneylenders and these give the appearance of exploiting poor and vulnerable people—they are a blight on our community. We appreciate the

council wants to attract businesses and see empty shops occupied. We do too. But this type of business is counter-productive and problematic. Before the riots there was a bookmaker near where *Paddy Power* wants to open, and there were always of crowds of people gathered outside, drinking and smoking. It was very intimidating. For the sake of a community which is still in shock from the riots and struggling to recover, we urge you to reject this application and focus on businesses which will lift the community, not suck the life out of it. (Nia Reynolds, West Croydon Community Association, speaking at the Croydon Licensing Sub-committee meeting, 5 March 2013)

Others objectors alleged connections between criminality, drugs, 'gang culture' and the presence of betting shops in the borough. These views, while noted, failed to convince the licensing sub-committee that the licence should be refused. As in the case of the licensing of Sexual Entertainment Venues, local authorities cannot take into account 'moral objections' to gambling and instead, must judge an application for a betting licence solely in relation to three key licensing objectives: preventing gambling being a source of crime and disorder, ensuring it's fair and open, and minimizing any risk to children and vulnerable people. In this instance, neither the pleas of the objectors nor the fact that *Paddy Power* already had a shop at 300 metres or so along the road were considered sufficient grounds for licence refusal (tellingly, there was no objection from local police). The betting shop opened in 2013, the seventh *Paddy Power* branch in Croydon.

This type of local campaign, like those against Sexual Entertainment Venues, is far from isolated, with similar instances across the country. But while there are only 180 or so lap dance clubs in Britain, there are well over 8000 betting shops (nearly 85% of these belonging to the 'Big 4'—*William Hill, Ladbrokes, Coral* and *Paddy Power*). While this number has probably halved from 1970, the visibility of these on local shopping streets like London Road has led to a widespread assertion there has been a major expansion in recent years, with betting shops taking over vacant or cheap properties at a time of recession. Some politicians suggest their constituencies are being 'swamped': Tottenham MP David Lammy argues betting shops are a 'parasite' on the High Street:

Betting shops are mushrooming across London and residents want to prevent them…There are more than 60 betting shops on Haringey's High Streets. Green Lanes has seven crammed into a 350m stretch of road; along the Tottenham High Road, there are another 13 … Our community is saturated with these gambling outlets, appearing in numbers far beyond what is needed to provide choice for consumers. The High Streets in my constituency are besieged with chains of betting shops, clustered together with hostile, tinted windows … Rival chains open up next door to each other to steal custom in areas known to be most profitable. Anyone on Green Lanes or the Tottenham High Road can tell you they are a haven for anti-social behaviour. Large numbers of men congregate outside these shops to smoke and drink, causing a nuisance and making an intimidating sight for residents. Police are often called to deal with abusive patrons. (Lammy 2014: np)

These are pretty serious allegations, and the language loaded. There's an adoption of hydraulic metaphors here, with our High Streets described as 'flooded' by a rising tide of betting shops. Like lap dance clubs, these are accused of coarsening the physical and moral character of the High Streets by attracting a disreputable male clientele. While the popularity of gambling is acknowledged, the rhetoric suggests there are more than enough to satisfy existing demand, with the tactics of the chains being to position their businesses in places where they can draw in new customers. The specific concern here is that the local state is powerless to stem the flow, with licensing and planning regulations insufficiently robust to prevent new betting shops opening. Even those who were pivotal in encouraging the liberalization of gambling under New Labour (via the *2005 Gambling Act* which transferred the licensing of gambling from magistrates courts to local authorities) concede municipal law is now insufficient to 'turn the tide'. For example, Harriet Harman, as Shadow Secretary for Culture, Media and Sports, and MP for Peckham, South London, has retrospectively criticized the introduction of the Gambling Act that she had previously voted for at each stage of its passage. As she explained in a Channel Four *Dispatches* investigation: 'If we had known then what we know now [*about the clustering of Betting Shops*], we wouldn't have allowed this, because it is not just ruining the High Street it is ruining people's lives'. Likewise, in a constituency report, she suggested 'the proliferation of bookmakers is damaging the look and feel of our High Streets, making them feel less safe and less welcoming, and making our High Streets less diverse' (Harman 2011:12).

But it's not only politicians and those with a vested interest in the fortunes of their local High Street who are concerned there are too many betting shops in town and city centres. In the surveys carried out by Populus for the Royal Society of Public Health (2015), 54% of 2050 respondents felt betting shops limit healthy choices, 52% think they have a poor impact on mental health and 49% that they play no role in promoting social interaction. Deloittes' (2013) research similarly suggested 52% wanted to see fewer betting shops on the High Street (cf. 31% who wanted fewer charity shops, and 16% who wanted fewer nail bars and beauty shops) while the ComRes survey for the Local Government Association (2012) revealed 50% feel that clusters of betting shops on the High Street have a negative impact on the vibrancy of the High Street (second only to sex shops and lap dance clubs, at 68%). In the same survey, 68% of 1875 surveyed stated it was wrong that a bank or other financial (A2) land use could be converted into a betting shop without seeking planning permission, and a quarter of 344 local authority planning officers questioned suggested there was already a problem with clusters of betting shops affecting the vibrancy and local economic development of the High Street. All this points to something of a social consensus that there are more than enough betting shops out there, with the emergence of new clusters deemed particularly worrying given the potential this has to damage the vitality and viability of High Streets, especially in 'struggling' areas.

So, in the hierarchy of 'unwanted land uses' on the High Street, the bookmaker or betting shop seems to be fairly near the top of the pile. Indeed, while Mary Portas' review of High Streets has very little to say about unwanted businesses like lap dance clubs, money lenders, fast food takeaways or tanning centres, it states unequivocally that 'the influx of betting shops, often in more deprived areas, is blighting our High Streets' (Portas 2011: 29). In turn, her report advocated a change to planning law to make it harder to convert retail shops units into betting shops by putting them into their own 'Use Class' so that policies could be brought in to limit their opening. Interestingly, this is in the same review arguing bingo is a good, old-fashioned community-based activity bringing people together in a lively, convivial manner, and deserves a comeback as a way of regenerating High Streets. Perhaps, this is because it's traditionally been regarded as an essentially feminized form of leisure, and one involving working-class women spending relatively petty sums (Bedford 2011). In contrast, betting shops have been depicted as frequented principally by men often staking—and potentially losing—more substantial amounts.

Such classed, and gendered, stereotypes begin to suggest why some forms of gambling appear more vilified than others. In terms of the current, and very vocal, opposition to betting shops, much of the blame for the rising anxiety appears to be related to the Fixed Odd Betting Terminals (FOBT) that now constitute around 50% of the profits of most betting shops. These are routinely depicted as the 'crack cocaine' of the gambling world, with opponents suggesting it's all-too-easy to lose hundreds of pounds in minutes. Images of an addicted working class hence abound, with the presence of gambling on the High Street viewed as particularly problematic when it occurs in areas where there are large numbers of relatively poor or unemployed men. Irrespective that the middle classes might gamble irresponsibly—albeit increasingly online—it's the poor who are regarded as vulnerable, and particularly susceptible, to the lure of the betting shop. Debt is depicted as a likely consequence, one that might trigger criminal or anti-social behaviour amongst disgruntled or desperate punters. The rhetoric here is akin to that of the nineteenth-century social reformers who argued that the working classes needed to be saved from the temptations of drink, gambling and other urban 'vices' in the interests of their health and productivity (Cunningham 1980). But is this equation of gambling and immorality really justified? And to what extent does it reveal anxieties about the visibility of working-class lifestyles in gentrifying cities? Noting the government strategies that have allowed gambling to penetrate ever-deeper into British life, in the remainder of this chapter I want to answer these questions, exploring the contradictions in attitudes towards gambling which have been brought into acute focus by the debates surrounding betting on the High Street.

Profiting from Poverty?

Given that it's now difficult to turn on the television without Ray Winstone literally shouting the odds at you, or *Paddy Power* courting controversy with one of its dubious taste adverts about Arab-owned football clubs or kicking cats up trees, it seems hard to believe betting was illegal away from sporting venues until the 1960s. But up to that decade the only way for people who were not attending a sporting event to lay bets was through turf accountants' 'runners' and illegal 'back street' bookies. However, recognition of the scale of unregulated betting on horse and greyhound racing, together with evidence that the working classes were capable of gambling 'with restraint' (Laybourn 2007) ultimately encouraged reform. The *1960 Betting and Gambling Act* hence repealed outdated legislation that forbade the use of any house, office or room for the purposes of betting, with the first advertised betting shops following in 1961. By the close of the decade there were as many as 16,000 betting shops in Britain. Initially, the majority were off the High Street, with a permit system allowing magistrates to determine location:

> Betting Shops were not to be situated on main roads, with side streets being considered more appropriate for this accepted but still dubious activity. Such shops were intended to be in shabby uninviting settings and the people that frequented them were not invited to linger there. The gambler was expected to slink furtively into the shop, shiftily place his/her bet and slide quietly out of the door, perhaps with an anxious glance over each shoulder. (Jones et al. 1994: 124)

The stipulation that all betting shops had to present 'dead windows', blacked out with little clue as to the nature of the business, was part of a deliberate attempt to ensure betting shops did not seduce or corrupt 'passers-by'. So too were the restrictions in terms of interior design, with betting shops spartan environments with little to encourage punters to dwell for long. However, the gradual liberalization of gambling laws in subsequent decades (e.g. amendments to the Gambling Act to allow live broadcast of races from 1984 onwards, limited evening opening from 1993 and Sunday opening from 1996) allowed the larger chains to innovate and thrive, with *William Hill, Ladbrokes, Coral* and *Mecca* (the latter eventually merging with *William Hill*) controlling 25% of the market by 1977 and 50% by the 1990s (Jones et al. 1994). Bold red, blue or green fronted-shops began to replace the more subdued betting shops of old.

In this context, the aforementioned *Gambling Act 2005* represented the most significant reform to gambling on the High Street since the 1960s, by allowing betting shops to openly advertise odds in their windows, at the same time it dispensed with the requirement that operators had to demonstrate local demand to secure licence for a new premises. But retrospectively, it appears the most important clauses of the *Gambling Act 2005* were those allowing up to four FOBT 'B2' gaming machines per licensed shop, typically, roulette machines with maximum bets of up to £100. The Gambling Commission suggested this was intended to limit the overall numbers of FOBT machines, but by 2011–12 there were around 32,000 such gaming machines operating, nearly double the 16,380 existing in 2006–07. Industry statistics suggest only around one in five who visit betting shops play these machines, but that the average spend per year for those who play machines is around four times more than that of the 'over the counter' gambler.

The introduction of FOBT machines has helped to retain a steady flow of customers in an era where over-the-counter betting on sports is declining relative to online gambling. The evidence—disputed though it is—suggests FOBT machines do not have great appeal for the 'traditional' punter who bets on sporting events but have actually pulled in a younger demographic that is not adverse to betting on sporting events but is most likely to play machines. But despite rhetoric to the contrary, there's been no major expansion in betting shops as a consequence: indeed, both *Ladbrokes* and *William Hill* both announced more closures than openings in 2014. Instead, the major consequence of changes in the sector (including the proliferation of FOTBs) appears to have been a concentration of chain bookmakers on the High Street, and the concomitant closure of stores in the inner city or neighbourhood centres, where footfall was not always sufficient to maintain viability. The fact that gambling seems 'recession proof' has proved significant here, with the appearance of voids on the High Streets providing new opportunities for bookmakers to identify prime frontages that would have previously been unaffordable, making their businesses more visible to more people, sometimes by opening multiple branches on a single High Street to maximize this exposure and compete with rival chains.

This increased visibility of betting shops appears to have consolidated the myth that betting shops are rapidly proliferating, with the idea that bookmakers are pursuing aggressive 'clustering' strategies, accepted as axiomatic. Anne Findlay and Leigh Sparks (2014a) quote from a *House of Commons* debate to suggest that this perceived clustering is a problem from multiple perspectives:

> This House is concerned that the clustering of betting shops in or close to deprived communities is being driven by increasing revenue from fixed odds betting terminals (FOBT) rather than traditional over the counter betting; believes that this has encouraged betting shop operators to open more than one premises in close proximity to one another; is aware of the growing concern in many communities about the detrimental effect this is having on the diversity and character of UK High Streets; is alarmed that people can stake as much as £100 every 20 seconds on these machines; is further concerned that the practice of single staffing in betting shops leaves staff vulnerable and deters them from intervening if customers suffer heavy losses thereby undermining efforts by the betting industry to protect vulnerable customers. (Clive Efford MP, *Hansard* Column 365, 8 Jan 2014)

It's worth quoting this at length, given—like the previously cited views of Harriet Harman, David Lammy et al.—it conflates a number of different arguments about betting shops and gambling in general. At least three separate arguments are mustered. The first is the idea that betting shops are pursuing a deliberative policy of locating their stores in deprived areas so they can profit from the desperation of the 'vulnerable' in society. Second is the contention that betting shops in disadvantaged areas attract anti-social behaviour, such as attacks on 'vulnerable staff'. Thirdly, it's argued that clustering is a particular problem, especially when this is on the High Street, because those who do not gamble are repelled by visible concentrations of betting shops. All of these arguments have their own logic, and are proving persuasive, but all demand further scrutiny.

The idea that betting shops prey on the poor is an argument that draws sustenance from the extensive evidence suggesting there are now more betting shops in poorer communities than in more affluent ones. For example, an impressively detailed geo-demographic analysis by Mark Astbury and Gaynor Thurstain-Goodwin (2007) for the Responsible Gambling Trust shows a correlation between gaming machine density, unemployment, deprivation and ethnic diversity. In a similar study, Heather Wardle et al. (2014) examined the characteristics of 386 'high-density machine zones', defined as those areas with significantly more than the average density of gaming machines. Labelling these 'risky places', they found 'a strong correlation between machine density and socio-economic deprivation' with high-density zones having 'higher income deprivation, more economically inactive residents and a younger population profile' (Wardle et al. 2014: 209). But while there's a correlation between localized deprivation and the presence of betting shops and gaming machines, it's an ecological fallacy to suggest that betting shops located in these areas prey exclusively on local, poorer residents. Indeed, analysis of customers' 'journeys-to-gamble' shows the majority actually travelled more than 3 km to bet, with the mean distance travelled being 25 km (Astbury and Thurstain-Goodwin 2007: Figure 67). Conversely, the British Gambling Prevalence Survey (2010) suggests that the unemployed are less likely to play machines in local bookmakers than in pubs or other venues (such as seaside arcades). Equally, it's worth noting those with managerial and professional occupations constitute 37% of slot machine players, and those with semi-routine jobs just 26%. The Health Survey for England (2012) confirms the prevalence of betting is actually lowest among the most deprived and highest amongst the wealthiest. This given, while betting, shops clearly rely on competitive presence, footfall and demand (like other High Street businesses) they do not appear to have any particular motivation for targeting the communities, where people are likely to have the least to spend (see Association of British Bookmakers 2014).

So, what of the alleged link between crime and gambling? This is certainly one that ties in nicely with the idea that betting shops target those in deprived communities. After all, the poor appear those least able to bear losses, and it's assumed they are more likely than more affluent gamblers to become indebted because of addiction to FOBT. The evidence for this assertion is patchy (e.g. the Health Survey England 2012, actually suggests those with no qualifications are less likely to be problem gamblers than those with higher education). Nonetheless, the fact that High Street betting shops are often close to pawn shops or payday loan-centres has been noted in some commentaries, which suggest this demonstrates some individuals are borrowing money at high rates of interest, or trading stolen goods to feed a gambling 'habit'. Others have even argued FOBT give some drug dealers a legitimate reason for carrying around large amounts of cash, with money laundering through betting shops mooted to be rife. This said, Gaynor Astbury and Mark Thurstain-Goodwin (2015) show there's virtually no difference between the number of crime events in town centres in general (10.09 per hectare) as opposed to areas within 400 m of a betting shop (10.48 per hectare). And a report commissioned by Ealing Council, with an eye to banning further betting shops in the Borough on the grounds of crime and disorder found that while there were more crime incidents associated with betting shops than most High Street uses, there were many fewer than around clubs or pubs, equivalent to one incident observed every eight hours or so. Noting the majority of these were low-level incidents unlikely to result in criminal charges, the conclusion was that there was no basis for justifying a new restrictive licensing policy— albeit it was stated 'clusters of licensed betting offices will give the impression of more of a problem to passers-by as it creates a "critical mass"' (cited in Ealing Licensing Committee minutes, 8 Nov 2012).

Despite this, the argument that the clustering of betting shops affects the vitality and viability of the High Street as a whole is one that enjoys considerable credibility (Fig. 7.1). Like the consumption of sexual entertainment, gambling retains a moral taint despite its legality, and continues to evoke images of contamination and corruption. And, like lap dance clubs or sex shops, betting shops are also accused of 'lowering the tone', and it this—as much as concern about crime, noise or nuisance— that seems to fuel attempts to limit their clustering. So, even though betting shops can obviously draw in customers, and provide much needed footfall on struggling High Streets, it's equally obvious they put off some, and potentially discourage other retail businesses from taking up vacant premises nearby. According to the Mayor of Hackney, Jules

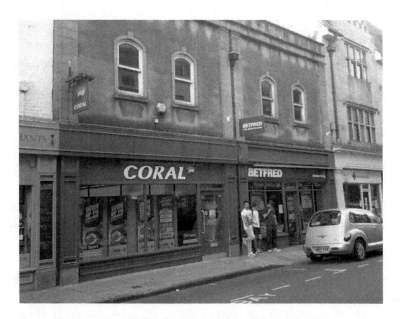

Fig. 7.1 A betting shop 'cluster' in Salisbury (photo: author)

Pipe, who made a submission to the government under the Sustainable Communities Act in 2014, 'clusters of betting shops' are 'sapping the vibrancy and variety from our High Streets, and squeeze out potential local enterprises which could use the premises for something positive and constructive' (cited in Cook 2014: np). This is a view mirrored by Mayor of London Boris Johnson (2011: np) who suggests 'betting shops have an important role to play in our culture and provide entertainment to many people' but that 'there's a balance to be struck between having betting shops as a part of the High Street retail mix and the negative impact they can have on shoppers and visitors when they start to dominate'.

But exactly what is a cluster? And how many betting shops does it take before the diversity of a High Street is irreparably damaged? These are difficult questions, especially when only around 4% of the total number of shops in Britain are betting shops, a figure that is much lower than the number of (for example) banks and estate agents which can be found next to one another on many British High Streets. Moreover, according to the Association of British Bookmakers (2014), in the inner city areas sometimes described as 'swamped' by betting shops, the proportion is typically less than this. For example, in Southwark—the first local authority to introduce new powers requiring planning permission for all new betting shops—the proportion was 2.3%, suggesting as few as 1 in 50 shops were betting shops. Is this really sufficient to undermine the vitality and viability of the High Street?

Regulating the Betting Shop

Whatever the reality of betting shops' impacts on the wider High Street environment, the argument that they need to be subject to tighter regulation has been vocal and sustained. Time and again, MPs and local councilors have argued for new controls to limit the 'spread' of betting shops. In some respects, these arguments have been disingenuous as there are a number of existing methods local authorities can use to influence the location and visibility of betting shops. Licensing—which, since the 1960s, has enacted a general principle of concealment in relation to gambling, keeping it away from areas where it's considered it might corrupt the young and vulnerable—provides the main technique of regulation here. Under the *Gambling Act 2005*, it's possible for licensing authorities to refuse or revoke licences when there's evidence of disorder being associated with a premises. But licensing is precautionary and forward-looking and not just reactive, meaning the evidence of the here-and-now can be discounted or downplayed with reference to a possible future (Hubbard 2015). This means betting shops can be refused licences if local authorities consider they could cause nuisance in the future by being located in unsuitable areas. Licensing policies can state this explicitly, and stipulate certain locations are unacceptable for gambling premises, such as those close to premises frequented by children or other vulnerable persons such as schools and parks. However, the presumption enshrined in the *Gambling Act 2005* is that betting shops are always acceptable unless there's clear evidence they might encourage crime and disorder, putting the onus on local authorities to prove otherwise. Given that bookmakers can usually employ licensing solicitors who are adept at persuading licensing committees, adequate measures will be put in place to restrict access to children, protect vulnerable persons and prevent crime and disorder, local authorities seem to be limited in their capacity to refuse licences to well-run, national chains.

It's here that local authorities have instead turned to planning control to try to prevent the opening of new premises. Like licensing, planning is ostensibly concerned only with valid material considerations (i.e. the visual appearance of a development, its impact on the setting and potential environmental nuisance), and not moral judgments about whether gambling makes a valuable contribution to society. But the *Town and Country Planning (Use Classes) Order 1987* makes it theoretically possible to prevent the conversion of existing retail uses into betting shops by suggesting that it constitutes a material change of use. In this categorization, betting shops fall within Class A2—which covers banks, estate agencies, building societies and other financial institutions—with any change in use between these not requiring planning permission (meaning a local authority cannot prevent a disused bank building being converted into a betting shop). In addition, it's permitted for Use Classes A3 (restaurants and cafés), A4 (drinking establishments) and A5 (hot food takeaways) to be converted to Class A2. However, converting an A1 retail shop to a betting shop always requires planning permission, and some local authorities have tried to make this difficult through policies citing detrimental impacts on the vitality and viability of the High Street as a possible reason for refusal. Many local authorities have stipulated the proportion of A2 frontages in a given town or local centre should not exceed a given threshold, typically 15–30%, claiming this is necessary to protect the 'active uses' on High Streets that 'create activity and interest directly related to passing pedestrians' (e.g. see Waltham Forest Development Management Policy DM26, 2013). However, some local authorities have gone further to argue that no more than three successive frontages in a retail area can be non-retail A2 use.

In theory, then, local authorities can prevent betting shops taking over retail units on High Streets on the basis this would create an imbalance between retail and non-retail. But in practice, when such policies have been tested at appeal they have often been found wanting. For example, after having been refused planning permission for two new betting shops in Waltham Forest, *Paddy Power* appealed successfully, with the Planning

Inspector ruling that these did not constitute 'a proliferation' and that the council's allegations of anti-sociality around existing betting shops lacked evidence given supermarkets, chemists and even the local library reported more crime than any of the existing betting shops (Independent Planning Inspector, APP/U5930/A/13/2204805, 19 Feb 2014). Other examples show that refusals based on notions of 'damaging clustering' can also be overturned. For example, in a case in Islington (V5570/A/12/2189530, 11 June 2013) the Inspector found 3–4% of units spread out over an area with a 500 m radius did not amount to an undue concentration of betting shops, and permitted the development contrary to local authority policy. Likewise, refusal of the conversion of disused chemist shop into a betting shop in Glossop was reversed at appeal with the inspector arguing this would 'not lead to a loss of vitality and viability of a shopping area' given the existing amount of non-retail use in the town centre was 'not high or damaging' (APP/H1033/A/12/2183093, 12 Dec. 2012). Even in cases where planning inspectors suggest it's not clear that a new betting shop will make 'an exceptionally valuable' contribution to vitality and viability, conversions from A1 to A2 have been allowed at appeal on the basis that it's better to have a betting shop than an empty premises. For example, in Rochdale town centre, where nearly a third of retail units were vacant at the time, the planning inspector argued a new betting shop would be 'securing a long term use, improving the appearance of the building … attracting customers to an area where there is currently little demand for retail units' (APP/P4225/A/14/2223506, 14 October 2014).

The fact that betting shop chains often emerge victorious from appeals confirms Sarah Blandy and Feng Wang's view (2013: 201) that successful corporate actors can 'usually ensure that legal and administrative discretion is exercised in their favour'. Irrespective, the judgments of planning inspectors cast doubt on the credibility of claims that betting shops are having particularly damaging impacts on High Streets. In a number of cases, inspectors have concluded that betting shops generate a higher level of footfall than some retail uses and that visits to them are often linked to trips to other shops and services. In one particularly well-publicized case, an appeal against Newham's refusal of planning permission for the change of use of a retail unit to a betting shop was upheld because the Council 'provided little detailed evidence to support its assertion that the proposal would detract from the health of local shopping centres' and offered no 'explanation of exactly what harm would be caused' (APP/ G5750/A/12/2168137, 10 May 2012). As Anne Findlay and Leigh Sparks (2014b: 310) argue, 'It's often contended that betting shops attract an unsavory clientele and that this puts other customers off … [*but*] this is not actually a planning issue but a policing and security issue'.

So even though the government has now made changes to the Use Classes Order making betting shops a 'sui generis' land use (i.e. outside the Use Classes Order, and no longer an A2 use), refusals of planning permission will not always be easy to defend. Likewise, mooted changes to local licensing policy, such as the introduction of Cumulative Impact Policies for betting shops (refusing any additional licences in 'saturated areas'), could also be defeated at judicial review. This is because, once moral prejudices about gambling are stripped away, it's very hard to demonstrate that the addition of one more betting shop to a High Street is likely to have any significant negative consequence, particularly in streets where there are vacant units present. Clearly, were the numbers of betting shops to begin to seriously unbalance the retail mix of the High Street, then the outcome might be different, but as it stands there's a good deal of evidence to suggest that a betting shop can attract significantly more customers than retail units of similar size, and that those using them combine their trips with shopping, complementing the main retail function of the High Street.

This said, the notion that betting shop customers contribute to the health and vibrancy of the High Street remains seriously hampered by stereotypes of 'the addicted class' (Welsh et al. 2014). This is unfortunate given the limited, but sustained, body of anthropological and sociological research suggesting gambling should not be understood solely in terms of an addiction paradigm, nor dismissed as irrational. For example, Mark Neal (2005) insists gambling is also about fun, conviviality, excitement, drama and escape. His observations about the different clientele encountered at different times of day in the typical British betting shop emphasizes this, given many trips are not about gambling large sums but enriching mundane routines of shopping, walking the dog or travelling to and from work. For example, he talks of 'weekday morning punters', whom he identifies as mainly male pensioners:

The morning was an important leisure part of the day for such men: it provided time-out from domestic arrangements; the visit itself was sociable, interesting and fun; and small-stake/high-yield bets provided them with an ongoing interest for the rest of the day. The benefits were not just restricted to their time in the shops, but were ongoing: the racing and betting became the subject of conversations with family and friends throughout the rest of the day; the multiple and pool bets provided a dream of riches that they could 'tap into' for the next few hours. For many such men, the trip to the betting shop was thus far from an isolated, irrational activity; it was highly sociable, and wholly understandable in terms of domestic, social and, indeed, financial, priorities. (Neal 2005: 296)

Continuing, Neal (2005) identifies other 'types': the lunchtime punter for whom a trip to the local shop was an integral part of the working day (particularly in dull or stressful jobs), the afternoon crowds, which can include large number of unemployed or homeless men who use the shops as *de facto* social centres, and the committed Saturday punters reveling in the busier, rowdier atmosphere engendered by the 'big races' shown at the weekend. In all cases, Neal argues these groups are gambling with no real expectation of winning. Rather, they expect to lose, and view this as the price they pay for participating in a (relatively accessible) form of leisure and sociality.

For sure, it's possible to visit betting shops and not regard them as particularly sociable, especially at times when there's only a solitary punter present or a few scattered round the room, some playing machines, others head down in copies of *The Racing Post* (Fig. 7.2). Often conversation is limited to brief 'banter' between staff and customers as bets are laid, or winnings picked up, and, save the inevitable sighs, expletives and expansive gestures of disappointment accompanying losses, few punters do much to attract comment. But, as Rebecca Cassidy (2014) shows, there's a sense of belonging and identity forged between customers, something the classification of punters into different 'types' can obscure. Visiting a betting shop binds participants into an imagined community, one that is resolutely masculine, has its roots in working-class culture and can be described, according to Cassidy, as anti-gentrification. In describing betting shops as masculine, Cassidy (2014: 176) is drawing attention not so much to the gender of the clientele, but the fact that the betting shop is experienced as a 'distinctively male place, with a set of rules that codify what men, and by implication, women, do, and should do'. As a space

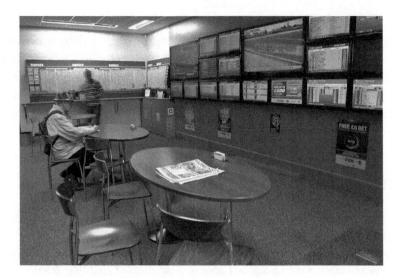

Fig. 7.2 A typical British betting shop interior (photo: author)

where particular (and arguably disappearing) notions of working-class masculinity can be performed and recast, largely out of the gaze of the women who exclude themselves from these settings, the betting shop provides a space where certain masculine traits are valued (e.g. an ambivalent, stoic attitude to loss, a privileging of calculation over instinct, and, more negatively, a degree of casual sexism).

All of this suggests that the efforts of regulators to crackdown on betting shops relies on the presentation of stereotypes of irrational masculine behaviour, stereotypes which draw sustenance from representations of residualized cultures badly out of step with those of the idealized, responsible consumer-gentrifier. Images of addicted, even dangerous, individuals abound. Empirical observations suggest this is far from the full picture. But even if it were the case that significant numbers of those frequenting betting shops are losing significant amounts of money on FOBT, Mark Whitehead et al. (2011) suggest that using planning and licensing regulation to tackle this issue by reducing the opportunities for the 'problem gambler' to access machines on the High Street is misguided, as gambling is deeply embedded in community life in the UK. Likewise, Gerda Reith (2013) argues there's a need for a more nuanced geopolitical interpretation of the distributions of gambling harms than one that figures this as a problem of 'flawed' consumers in 'vulnerable' communities. Using myths of addiction as a way of positioning betting shops as having a negative impact on vitality and viability of the High Street is then a questionable tactic. In this sense, representing betting shops as less valuable to High Streets than, for example, shops, banks, or estate agents seems to betray class-based prejudices against what is ultimately an affordable and popular form of sociality and leisure.

References

Association of British Bookmakers. (2014). *The truth about betting shops.* London: ABB.

Astbury, G., & Thurstain-Goodwin, M. (2015). *Contextualising machine gambling characteristics by location.* London: Responsible Gambling Trust.

Bedford, K. (2011). Getting the bingo hall back again? Gambling law reform, economic regeneration and the gendered limits of "casino capitalism". *Social and Legal Studies, 20*(3), 369–388.

Blandy, S., & Wang, F. (2013). Curbing the power of developers? Law and power in Chinese and English gated urban enclaves. *Geoforum, 47,* 199–208.

British Gambling Prevalence Survey. (2010). *British Gambling Prevalence Survey.* London: Gambling Commission.

Brooks, G. (2012). Challenging the myth of urban regeneration: Raising the profile of problem gambling with a media campaign. *Journal of Gambling Studies, 28*(4), 741–751.

Cassidy, R. (2014). 'A place for men to come and do their thing': Constructing masculinities in betting shops in London. *The British Journal of Sociology, 65*(1), 170–191.

Cook, B. (2014). More calls for betting shop limits. *Local Government Chronicle,* 26 February, http://www.lgcplus.com/news/more-calls-for-betting-shop-limits/5068427.article

Cunningham, H. (1980). *Leisure in the industrial revolution, 1780–1880.* New York: St Martin's Press.

Deloitte. (2013). *The future of the British remote betting and gaming industry.* London: Deloitte.

Department of Culture, Media and Sport. (2002). *A safe bet for success.* London: DCMS.

Findlay, A., & Sparks, L. (2014a). High Streets and town centres policy. In N. Wrigley & E. Brookes (Eds.), *Evolving High Streets: Resilience and reinvention*. ESRC/University of Southampton.

Findlay, A., & Sparks, L. (2014b). Unlucky No. 13? *Town and Country Planning*, *83*(8), 308–311.

Greater London Authority. (2012). *Croydon opportunity area planning framework*. London: GLA.

Greater London Authority. (2014). *London town centre health check analysis report*. London: GLA.

Harman, H. (2011). The problem of betting shops blighting High Streets and communities in low income areas. London, House of Commons. Retrieved from http://www.harrietharman.org/uploads/d2535bc1-c54e-6114-a910-cce7a3eff966.pdf

Health Survey England. (2012). *Health survey for England*. London: HMSO.

Hubbard, P. (2015). Law, sex and the city: Regulating sexual entertainment venues in England and Wales. *International Journal of Law in the Built Environment*, *7*(1), 5–20.

Johnson, B. (2011). Mayor calls for planning controls over betting shop boom. https://www.london.gov.uk/media/mayor-press-releases/2011/10/mayor-calls-for-planning-controls-over-betting-shop-boom

Jones, P., Hillier, D., & Turner, D. (1994). Back street to side street to High Street: The changing geography of betting shops. *Geography*, 122–128.

Lammy, D. (2014). Unite against betting shops and we can beat this High Street parasite. Tottenham Journal, 19 March, http://www.tottenhamjournal.co.uk/news/comment_unite_against_betting_shops_and_we_can_beat_this_high_street_parasite_1_3453499

Laybourn, K. (2007). *Working-class gambling in Britain c. 1906–1960s: The stages of the political debate*. Lewiston, NY: Mellen Press.

Neal, M. (2005). 'I lose, but that's not the point': Situated economic and social rationalities in horserace gambling. *Leisure Studies*, *24*(3), 291–310.

Portas, M. (2011). The Portas review: An independent review into the future of our High Streets. http://www.maryportas.com/news/2011/12/12/the-portas-review/

Reith, G. (2013). Techno economic systems and excessive consumption: A political economy of 'pathological' gambling. *The British Journal of Sociology*, *64*(4), 717–738.

Royal Society of Public Health (2015). *Health on the High Street*. London: RSPH.

Townshend, T. G. (2016). Toxic High Streets. Journal of Urban Design, online early, doi:10.1080/13574809.2015.1106916

Wardle, H., Keily, R., Astbury, G., & Reith, G. (2014). 'Risky places?': Mapping gambling machine density and socio-economic deprivation. *Journal of Gambling Studies, 30*(1), 201–212.

Welsh, M., Jones, R., Pykett, J., & Whitehead, M. (2014). The "Problem Gambler" and socio-spatial vulnerability. In F. Gobet & M. Schiller (Eds.), *Problem gambling: Cognition, prevention and treatment*. Palgrave: Basingstoke.

Whitehead, M., Jones, R., & Pykett, J. (2011). Governing irrationality, or a more than rational government? Reflections on the rescientisation of decision making in British public policy. *Environment and Planning A, 43*(12), 2819.

8

Fast Food, Slow Food

Debates on morality and value are never far away in discussions of High Street trends. Witness, for example, the now established critiques of 'fast fashion', in which cheap, mass-produced goods arrive on the High Street courtesy of globalized production systems. As numerous commentators have highlighted (e.g. Crewe 2008; Tokalti 2008; Hoskins 2014), this involves mass market retailers such as *Primark* and *New Look* treading the path of least resistance, using cheap offshore labour to produce styles that are available on the High Street merely weeks after their initial exposure on the catwalks of Milan, Paris and New York. But there's a notable reaction against this, with the growing discontent with this type of model encouraging some consumers to seek an alternative in the form of 'slower' fashion. This takes different forms, from searching through thrift stores and charity shops for recycled bargains (Gregson et al. 2002) through to supporting fair trade and craft production, knitting and sewing (Crewe 2016). Arguably, the negativity surrounding fast fashion has also valorized clothes that are well-crafted, durable and of known provenance, with those that can afford it spending considerable sums on goods that they think are more ethical than those found in many High Street retailers (Crewe 2016).

© The Editor(s) (if applicable) and The Author(s) 2017
P. Hubbard, *The Battle for the High Street*,
DOI 10.1057/978-1-137-52153-8_8

This chapter suggests that many of these trends are mirrored—and even accentuated—in the geographies of the foodscape. Food and drink are by its very nature designed to be consumed relatively quickly, so some of the debates about durability do not necessarily apply: nevertheless, there are commonalities in the ways that cheap, mass-produced convenience purchases are represented as both socially and environmentally damaging. As we will see, in contemporary Britain, the discoursing of 'fast food' as dirty and ugly draws sustenance from a further set of concerns that are not so much about its environmental and social cost as its impact on the health of those who consume it. Those who buy fast food are not just stigmatized for consuming in an unethical manner, but showing scant regard for their own well-being, risking ill health and obesity. In contrast, those who shun fast food in favour of more 'ethical' alternatives, such as local, organic or craft products, are seen to be healthy, morally righteous consumers, demonstrating respect for themselves and the world around them. Given the force of narratives suggesting slow food is good, and fast food bad, it's hard to argue with such categorization. But, as always on the High Street, the value, worth and cost of our purchases is arguably not as clear-cut as we might initially suppose, and it's important to question how ideas of moral and ethical consumption are shaped by assumptions about class which are inevitably tipped in favour of the wealthy.

Fast Food Nation

It's clear that one of the most controversial businesses on the High Street is, perversely, also one of the most popular. At a time when many shops have struggled, and vacant units increased in number, 'fast food' takeaways have continued to proliferate. Maguire et al. (2015) estimate there has been a 50% increase in their number over the last two decades, with an 8% increase in 2009 alone (Thompson 2009). Chains including *McDonalds*, *Domino's Pizza* and sandwich store *Subway* have all continued to expand, with the latter increasing its number of outlets to over 2000 by 2015, but the vast majority of outlets remain independently owned. While no one seems able to provide reliable data about trends in this rapidly changing sector, there appears to be a shift away from what are regarded as traditional 'British' forms of hot food takeaway—especially the fish and chip shop—towards other forms of fast food, including those associated with recent in-migration. *McDonalds Allegra* (2009) focus on a 'typical' city to illustrate this, reporting that between 1978 and 2008 in Coventry, the number of fish and chip shops dropped from 61 to 31, at the same time the total number of fast food outlets increased from 27 to 141. While the latter included a wide variety of Turkish kebab stores, Chinese, Bangladeshi and Indian takeaways, and pizza outlets, a notable development was the growth in fried chicken shops, which grew 36% between 2003 and 2008, significantly outstripping growth for the fast food sector as a whole. There's now one chicken shop for every 1280 people in England, and one for every 1000 Londoners (*Greater London Authority* 2012). Although there's a perception such outlets have emerged to cater mainly for the inebriated, being thoroughly integrated with the night-time economy (Chap. 5), the growing popularity of relatively cheap, spicy fried chicken among those of school age appears significant here, especially in multi-cultural inner city contexts where outlets using halal meat are popular lunchtime venues for those from black and Asian families.

Despite this recent increase in takeaway numbers, the presence of fast food on our High Streets has always been controversial. For example, in the 1980s and 1990s, it was not uncommon to see local residents campaigning against *McDonalds* stores in British towns and cities (encouraging a short-lived national *Burger Off!* campaign). For some, these new franchised stores represented an unacceptable Americanization of the High Street, with 'McDonaldization' taken to represent the triumph of predictable, formulaic corporate culture over a more 'authentically' British way of dining (and shopping). In many senses, these protests were a reaction to the principles that underpin the proliferation of *McDonalds* and the other chains following in its wake (e.g. *KFC*, *Burger King*, *Pizza Hut*): as Ritzer (2003) has famously described, efficiency, calculability, predictability, and control have been the cornerstone of *McDonalds*' success, their appeal for consumers being that they offer both convenience and affordability. Critiques of 'fast food culture' hence focus on this appeal to rationality, with alarmist accounts seeing the dominance of fast food chains as symptomatic of the relentless speeding up of everyday life, with routines of family dining, as well as the natural rhythms of the body, being overwhelmed by the pace of modern urban life (Jabs and Devine 2006). For a Marxist humanist like Henri Lefebvre, the rise of fast food culture in his native France appeared to represent a 'flattening' of space and time, the triumph of abstract space and the imposition of a logic of exchangeability (Merrifield 2006). For Lefebvre, the fast food restaurant appeared the antithesis of the type of eating he thought best exemplified the warm, creative elements of human life: the traditional village festival (*la fête*), with its spontaneous and collective celebration of the local and distinctive. In contrast, *McDonalds* offers an 'abstract' form of food, signifying the colonization of space by capital. No wonder fast food restaurants feature so prominently in anti-globalist discourse: in Marc Augé's (1995) influential account of the 'super-modern' condition, they are described as the quintessential non-place, a symptom of anonymous globalization that is oddly comforting because of its ubiquity, but is ultimately alienating.

But it's not only local identity seen to be at the mercy of fast food culture. Down the years, numerous social movements have accused the fast food chains of perpetuating unsustainable farming practices and overwhelming local food production systems. Intense food production, low-wage economics, genetically modified crops, abuses of animal welfare, climate change: all have, to a lesser or greater degree, been pinned on transnational fast food conglomerates (Hughes 1995; McMichael et al. 2007). It's these anxieties about fast food cultures that have arguably taken new, exaggerated forms against the backdrop of growing concerns about obesity in the UK, encapsulated in the 2008 *Healthy Weight, Healthy Lives* strategy issued by the Department of Health to guide strategy across governmental departments. In the words of the strategy:

> Our vision for the future is one where the food that we eat is far healthier, with major reductions in the consumption and sale of unhealthy foods, such as those high in fat, salt or sugar, and all individuals choosing to eat levels of fruit and vegetables in line with recommended amounts consistent with good health. Individuals and families will have a good understanding of the impact of diet on their health, and will be able to make informed choices about the food they consume, with extra support and guidance for

those who need help. The food, drink and other related industries will support this through clear and consistent information, doing all they can to make food healthy. (Department of Health 2008: xiii)

Amongst talk of an 'obesity time-bomb', with one-third of children identified as overweight, and two-thirds of adults, the emphasis in this report was not so much about promoting exercise, but encouraging healthy lifestyles by 'nudging' consumers towards healthier consumption choices (see Evans and Colls 2009, on public health pedagogy in Britain). Reinforcing this vision, the Strategy called local authorities to use existing planning powers to control the number and location of fast food outlets, suggesting that reducing the availability of certain foods on the High Street would encourage people to consume differently. This narrative has been echoed in numerous missives from diverse think tanks and public health organizations. For example, at the United Kingdom Public Health Association Annual Forum in 2009 the 'Food & Nutrition special interest group' pledged to work to 'embed in planning processes the ability of local communities to grow, sell and buy locally produced food' insisting 'local authorities should use their restrictive powers (by-laws) to create these opportunities by restricting fast food outlets' (cited in Caraher et al. 2013).

In a context where a *OnePoll* survey in 2014 suggested the average UK consumer eats as many as 84 'fast food' meals per year, and at least one-third of the average household food budget goes on takeaways and restaurant meals, this desire to discourage the consumption of often high fat, high salt foods by clamping down on takeaways seems sensible. This is particularly so when these often-cheap takeaways often appear 'clustered' in the proximity of schools, tempting pupils to spend their dinner money on food that, to teenage tastebuds, is eminently more tasty than school meals, and is often more affordable. The national media has often highlighted this phenomenon, with a search to find the 'worst' culprit leading several High Streets to be crowned Britain's 'fast food mile'. *The Daily Mirror* has suggested this is West Green Road, in Haringey, London— with '10 fried chicken shops, six kebab shops, seven greasy spoon cafés and an array of Chinese and Caribbean takeaways all undercutting school canteen prices' (Cookney 2014: np)—but Gloucester's Eastgate and Levenshulme's Stockport Road (Manchester) have elsewhere been described in similar terms. But many other local shopping streets appear equally unbalanced: just outside Southampton University, and near to two primary and one secondary school, Burgess Road is devoted to fast food and 'grab and go' consumption, with no less than 17 takeaways, discount bakers (including *Greggs*, boasting a £2 lunch deal of pasty and drink) or burger restaurants within 500 m of one another (Fig. 8.1). In such locations, we are told fast food takeaways are 'vultures circling round schools', tempting the young into unhealthy eating practices. Even in the midst of the Easter vacation I note one window boasting a 'Back 2 School' special—one piece of chicken, two chicken nuggets, onion rings and fries for £2.50.

In the discourses talking of 'toxic' High Streets, arguments have hence been arrayed to suggest fast food outlets need to be discouraged, particularly around schools. These are beginning to persuade local authorities

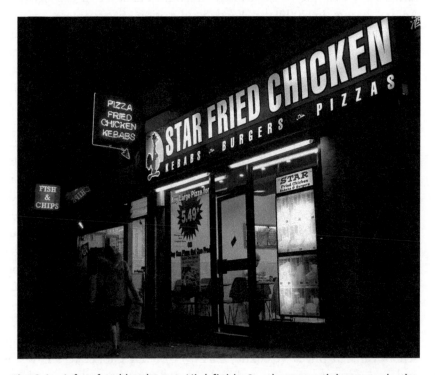

Fig. 8.1 A fast food landscape, Highfields, Southampton (photo: author)

of the need for action: in 2009, Waltham Forest Borough Council became the first to effectively ban takeaways selling hot food near schools through policies suggesting planning permission would not be given for any within 400 metre of schools. Here the logic deployed is that few school pupils are prepared to walk more than 400 metres (around five minutes' walk) to purchase lunch, a principle now informing the policies of many other local authorities. For example, Britain's largest local authority, Birmingham City Council, adopted a similar 400 metre guideline in 2013 in its Supplementary Planning Document for Shopping and Local Centres. Simultaneously, it introduced regulations refusing planning permission for hot food takeaways in shopping areas where currently more than one in ten units are already food outlets, resulting in the refusal of 15 applications in the first two years of its enforcement. Some local authorities have imposed even stricter limits: for instance, the Plymouth Plan (2012), suggests a maximum of 5% of units in any given shopping streets can be a hot food takeaway.

Such planning restrictions are defended primarily with reference to the need to create healthier High Streets, but there's also frequent allusion in policy documents to noise, smell, litter and neighbourhood aesthetics. Takeaways have been criticized for being detrimental to environmental amenity as well as local well-being:

> Local people want government to give councils the powers to tackle unsightly clusters of … takeaways that can blight so many of our High Streets. People want action so the places they live, work and shop can be revitalised to reflect how they want them to look and feel. Councils want High Streets to thrive and are on the side of local people and are ready to put a stop to high numbers of unsavoury takeaways … where there is a demand to do so. High Streets across the UK have suffered a cardiac arrest and it's now time to let local authorities step in and deliver the necessary life support. (Cockell, cited in Carpenter 2012: np)

This conflation of environmental and health concerns is significant, showing aesthetic and moral considerations often collide in judgments of what 'fits' on the High Street. Here, the bold, bright signage of many fast food takeaways is interpreted as garish and gaudy, and the smells emanating from inside malodorous. There's also much made of the fact that 'food on the go' is the 'cause' of significant amounts of litter (DEFRA 2004). But, somewhat oddly, reference to hot food takeaways generating such nuisances is routinely made in reports which provide data only on the connections between fast food and obesity (e.g. *Public Health England* 2014; Burgoine et al. 2014).

So, while policies aiming to reduce the numbers of fast food restaurants on our High Streets sound eminently sensible given the assumed connection between obesity and the proliferation of eateries selling 'bad food', opposition to fast food restaurants goes beyond a mere preoccupation with healthy eating to encompass wider anxieties about the moral geography of the contemporary foodscape. Arguably, these concerns betray both class- and race-based anxieties. Fast food is, from the perspective of opponents, not just unhealthy, but its relative cheapness is equated with vulgarity and uncleanliness. Take, for example, this description of chicken shops in a *Guardian* article focused on the employment of immigrant labour in London's takeaways:

> At *Fat Chaps* (*Best Turkish Cuisine*), a middle-aged man from Uzbekistan is serving chips over the counter; the air hangs heavy with the smell of frying, and the floor is slippery with grease. A sign behind him reads: "Please do not ask for credit as a smack in the mouth often offends" … At *Mighty Chicken & Ribs*, at around midnight, the extractor fan is not working, the tables are unwiped and grimy, and rubbish is exploding from the bin. The only member of staff on duty, a student from Pakistan, is also unable to give precise details about his pay arrangements, and claims not to know how to contact his employer. Inspectors tell him off for leaving a half-eaten burger (his supper) behind the till and for storing the chicken on top of the bread in the freezer, along with the day's takings (wrapped in a plastic bag). "You can't keep money in the freezer." Border Agency staff check his student visa, which they report is about to expire. (Gentleman 2012: np)

In this, and many similar reports, there's an obvious stereotyping of immigrant-run takeaways as dirty and disordered, propping up racist imaginaries in which black and ethnic minorities are understood to be a threat to the sanctity and cleanliness of the nation. In many senses, this undermines more positive constructions of ethnic entrepreneurship on the High Street (e.g. Hall 2011), and the pleas of the *New Economics*

Foundation (2003) that we should cherish small-scale retail livelihoods. Indeed, takeaways represent one of the few sectors on the High Street where chains are actually depicted as preferable to independently run outlets: in a report on the link between chicken shops and poor diet, Shift (2012: 6) suggest the latter are significantly more likely to serve meals with high calorific content as they use 'unsophisticated cooking techniques' and oil of a low standard, often rich in saturated and trans-fats.

The independent chicken shop or takeaway, even more so than the fast food chains, consequently invokes a set of myths about the demise of the 'British' High Street, the 'British' diet, and even the 'British' way of life. These modern fears and anxieties hence need to be understood in the light of sedimented myths and rituals of eating in Britain. Norbert Elias' (1982) figurational analysis of manners and civility reminds us these are not constant, with the boundaries of polite consumption shifting markedly over time. In Britain, we have become arguably much more casual in our eating practices, and present generations are much more prone to snack than their parents were. In a 'fast paced' society, eating alone has become much more the norm. Yet some constants remain, with social relationships of friends and family still cemented, and celebrated, by 'eating together' (Marshall 2005). 'Calendrical' meals—e.g. a trip to a restaurant for someone's birthday or a summer BBQ get-together—are a particularly important way of performing family identity as well as providing an opportunity to display one's taste and distinction to others, but this can be extended to daily breakfast, lunch and dinner, all of which are idealized as social occasions for catching up with housemates, friends or colleagues. In contrast, 'food on the go' is still seen as essentially asocial, something one consumes when one is hungry, a giving in to basic 'stomach' needs. Kebabs, chips and chicken takeaways remain culturally devalued, and even vilified, depicted as something bought when one is drunk and hungry, coming back from a club, or on the way to a football match, for example. Gill Valentine (1998: 161) suggests 'to eat in the street is to give in to animal urges: it has connotations of primitiveness, bestiality, the wild … to eat on the street is to graze, to use hands rather than cutlery, to threaten social rules concerning the use of the mouth: to lick, chew noisily'. Hot food takeaways are not refined, and eating them can be a messy business, especially on the move.

Gnawed bones, flakey pasty crumbs, and discarded greasy wrappers on the pavements are then presented as a consequence of the rise of a new breed of fast food premises that are exploitative, low-wage and unhygienic. It is an example of how cheap or affordable food can become associated with dirt, triggering certain disgust reactions. Is it this, as much as concerns about obesity, which inform governmental policies, designed to limit fast food on our High Street? At times, it appears so. Certainly, when the Coalition government threatened a tax on all takeaway foods sold at 'above ambient temperature' in 2012, a storm was kicked up with a number of commentators accusing them of imposing a 'cornish pasty' tax that would effectively push up the price of 'ordinary people's food'. Despite the government's decision to back down in this instance, the general vilification of fast food takeaways, chicken shops, and 'grab and go' snack retailers remains in marked contrast to the cultural celebration of local produce, real coffee and 'slow' food, all of which are actively promoted in visions of the good High Street.

The Rise of Foodie Culture

Many of the key ethical questions of our time relate to food: as well as the aforementioned obesity panic, questions of animal welfare and the prosperity of small-scale food producers, our consumption choices are innately related to questions of what is socially just and ecologically sustainable. The answers to these questions are of course difficult, and highly contested, but at times, they are presented as straightforward. Indeed, sometimes the divide between 'good' and 'bad' food appears sharply drawn. Fruit and vegetables are good, food rich in saturated fats, salt and refined sugar bad. Fast food, alongside convenience, packaged foods, is seen as especially bad and considered an unethical choice when compared to fruits or vegetables that have been locally sourced or organically grown. Dairy, meat and fish are more problematic, but given that they can be a source of protein and vitamins, these are generally regarded as an essential part of a good diet, so long as they are sustainably produced. But contradictions abound. We are told to buy British, but what does this mean in an era when supermarket-bought 'Scottish salmon' might have been sourced in Norway, and merely smoked in Scotland, or when some supermarkets sell New Zealand lamb shanks in misleading packaging suggesting they are actually British? And while some fish are identified as sustainable, what if those fish are intensively farmed, or caught using methods regarded as problematic in animal welfare terms?

These questions place the onus firmly onto the consumer, requiring us to scrutinize our food choices, becoming knowledgeable about where our food is coming from, what nutritional value it has and the best way of preparing it. As Kneafsey et al. (2008) emphasize, this is often discoursed as requiring a 'reconnection' between producers and consumers. Fast and packaged food reveals little or nothing of its origins, leading to suspicion it must be produced in unethical, inequitable ways that damage societies and environments alike. 'Good food', in contrast, needs to be found and sourced appropriately. And to guide us in this task, the media provides us with a plethora of websites, TV programmes and broadsheet supplements. Celebrity chefs—Jamie, Rick, Hugh and the like—provide some of our key reference points here, encouraging us to forge new relationships with the food we eat, shop more sensibly, grow our own vegetables, be discerning in the way we cook. In keeping with the mood of austerity nostalgia, the rhetoric is one that abhors waste—take, for example, Gregg Wallace's BBC series *Eat Well for Less*, which encouraged families to cook food from raw ingredients rather than buying ready-made meals—and it's also one values as 'traditional' working-class fare. But despite the emergence of this somewhat backward looking and thrifty culinary culture, which has revalued 'good, old-fashioned' dishes like pie and mash, there's a consistent accent on quality, provenance and 'authenticity' that provides a basis for the cultivation and display of a 'foodie' disposition. This, as Blythman (2010: 6) ascerbically observes, plays into the hands of a new gastronomic elite (gastronauts?) who 'live in lofts and stylish townhouses or in covetable country houses and hollyhock cottages' and are so obsessed with caramelizing crème brûlées perfectly 'they give each other blow torches for Christmas'.

Contemporary foodie culture is then promoted through a peculiar mix of pre-emptive health advice (suggesting poor diet is the prime cause of obesity) and representations showing the pleasure that can be derived from preparing 'real' food from basic ingredients (via self-sufficient 'veg patch capitalism'). For instance, Lucy Potter and Claire Westall (2013) focus on the BBC's *Great British Bake Off*, and its predecessor *The Great British Menu*, identifying these as attempts to encourage consumers to buy into a seemingly wholesome lifestyle and imagined culinary authenticity embedded within specific localities, food products and cookery techniques. Here, localist discourse is loaded with the 'moral and nostalgic' implications of home economy (Potter and Westall 2013: 169). David Bell and Joanne Hollows (2011) similarly describe Hugh Fearnley-Whittingstall's home-spun *River Cottage* series, and his 'campaigning culinary documentary' *Hugh's Chicken Run*, as examples of 'lifestyle programming' given they legitimate the tastes and dispositions associated with particular class factions. In these series, Hugh combines home-grown produce from his cottage garden with locally sourced meat and fish tracked down at Farmer's Markets across the South West, generously sharing the meals he prepares with friends and family in convivial surroundings. The tone is not preachy, but there's an implicit message that convenience food is not just lazy, but unhealthy and immoral.

The media's 'moralization of convenience food' (Jackson and Viehoff 2016) is widely apparent, with *Jamie's School Dinners* providing another case in point. This Channel Four series was justified as an attempt to improve school meals and do away with mass-produced water-injected turkey 'twizzlers' and chips, but was arguably also part of a broader school–based 'food pedagogy', casting a critical eye over the content of children's lunchboxes, and suggesting it was 'easy' for parents to pack a nutritious lunch box for their child. The parents of children sent to school with packed lunches low in vitamins and nutrition were condemned not for their lack of wealth per se but their lack of care. In this programme, feeding one's children cheap, processed food was taken to demonstrate a 'lack of taste, education and morality' (Pike and Leahy 2012: 436). Although convenience food can help time-poor parents cater to the tastes and dietary preferences of different family members (Jackson and Viehoff 2016), in this programme they were made to feel guilty for 'cheating', and accused of promoting unhealthy eating practices. But this is not the only example: at the extreme, the portrayal of parents allowing their children to eat 'junk' food has been vicious. Famously, when Rawmarsh secondary school in Rotherham converted its menu to healthier options, two mothers passed the pupils burgers and chips through the school railings at lunchtime because the new food was unpopular with their children. Consequently, the town was described as 'a place where fat stupid mothers fight for the right to raise fat stupid children' (Hattersley 2006: 24), parts of the media deploying a language barely concealing disgust for working class, 'obese' maternal bodies. As Peter Jackson (2016) argues, such examples provide plentiful evidence of the way social anxieties about food and diet spill over into a range of other concerns about regional stereotypes, gender and particularly class.

The imperatives around 'eating well' hence carry powerful moral overtones about how individuals ought to behave (Rich 2011). As such, while distinctions of good and bad food are obviously refracted through understandings of healthy, green and organic consumption (Slocum 2007), there remains considerable disgust projected onto those who appear reliant on convenience and fast food, a disgust Rachel Colls (2007) argues centres on the 'moral failings' of gluttony and sloth (see also Highmore 2008 and Rhys-Taylor 2013 on 'alimentary pedagogy'). However, this is rarely discussed in terms of the material constraints which restrict the choices of the less affluent: instead, there's a privileging of the values of the *petite bourgeoisie* which, explicitly or otherwise, render other people's 'lifestyle choices' as less legitimate and less 'ethical' (Bell and Hollows 2011). The shift in foodie culture away from gourmet appreciation of 'fine dining' towards 'ethical' or so-called *slow* consumption has been decisive here, and is reflected in some High Streets in the emergence of outlets dedicated to organic, fresh produce. In times gone by, these might have been described as alternative, hippy or countercultural food stores, but today they are more likely discoursed as local, 'community stores', even if the goods they sell are often sourced overseas. Such stores are set up as the antithesis of the supermarket, favouring shabby chic and rustic interiors rather than the brightly lit aisles that have become the 'paradigm of the everyday experience of modernisation' (Everts and Jackson 2009: 921). They are a clear reaction to the emergence of a global foodscape based on predictability and replication: in contrast to the supermarket, where brands seek to convey quality through design, images, and text, these new stores imbue their produce with authenticity primarily through the proprietor, a 'local' entrepreneur who is typically viewed as a source of trustworthy information about the origins and quality of produce (Everts and Jackson 2009). The design of the shop is thus not insignificant, creating an atmosphere in which the interaction between customer and owner is bequeathed with meaning and authenticity. Whitstable High Street—Britain's leading 'home town' (New Economics Foundation 2010)—boasts many examples, from a specialist in British cheese that sells hay-baked camembert (*The Cheese Box*), a deli specializing in Spanish and Italian goods, as well as English cheeses from Neal's Yard dairy (*David Brown Delicatessen*), the celebrated *Windy Corner Stores*, which sells locally produced no-yeast slow-fermentation artisanal bread, and *Waltshaw's Kentish Pantry* with its impressive range of free-range meat and eggs from local farms, local wet fish, coffee from the Canterbury micro-roastery and Kentish craft beers. Most of these shops encourage tasting, and sell platters that can be consumed at the counter or at some of the chairs and tables that appear at weekends when it's nice enough to sit outside.

Long marginalized by the modern supermarket, the grocery store is then undergoing a resurgence, and not solely for nostalgic reasons. Rather, grocery stores and wholefood delis allow consumers to engage with trusted individuals who promise to connect them to broader circuits of foodie culture by introducing them to local brands or specialties sourced further afield. In contrast to the relentless homogeny of *McDonalds*, *Tesco*, *Costa* and *Subway*, these promote local distinctiveness and sense of place. Slow food is integral to the creation of slow cities, places embracing eco-gastronomy and local produce in the interests of attracting consumers and tourists (Knox 2005). My home town of Faversham, for example, boasts a range of locally owned coffee shops and eateries that have prospered in recent times, with a newly minted Faversham Food Festival added to the pre-existing asparagus weekend, cherry festival and the annual hop-festival to produce a 'taste of Kent' brand vigorously promoted by the tourist authorities. In this respect, when *Costa* coffee applied to open in a disused shoe shop on the historic market place, there was a slew of opposition from local business owners who felt this would damage the town's emerging foodie reputation. For example, the owner of *Jittermugs* Fair Trade café and tapas shop—an intimate little shop themed around classic literature—went on record to suggest that 'a chain coffee shop will suck the life out of independent businesses and they won't be bringing in anything different ...When we started, we brought something different to Faversham. They are just the same as the other two in the big three—*Nero*, *Costa* and *Starbucks*. It's such a shame' (cited in Browning 2014: np). In the wake of hundreds of letters of objection, *Costa* withdrew their planning application. A year on, the vacant shop unit they were going to occupy remained vacant, but in the same period one of the local pubs was rebranded as a champagne and oyster bar, and the local farm shop began an ambitious £5m expansion plan to triple its floorspace.

But this revival is far from ubiquitous. Not every town can sustain the type of micro-eateries and specialty grocery stores found in a foodie oasis like Faversham or Whitstable (or some of the other small towns noted as centres of 'cuisine tourism', like Totnes, Hebden Bridge, Ludlow or Padstow). In many towns, aside from the supermarkets, the only alternative source of fresh meat, fish, fruit and vegetables is a weekly street market where, traditionally, stalls selling food and drink sat cheek by jowl with those specializing in second-hand books and DVDs, hosiery, cheap imported toys, fabrics, and assorted *bric a brac* from house clearances. Sophie Watson and David Studdert's (2006) suggest that these have been significant not only as a source of affordable food but also in terms of providing a space of sociality, where people from various backgrounds learn to get by and get along:

> Markets can offer possibilities not only for local economic growth but also for people to mingle with each other and become accustomed to each others' differences in a public space; in this way, markets can act as potential focal points for local communities. As sites of public interaction and retail spaces, where traders pay rent for their stalls, they could in some senses be described as public/private spaces, disrupting the often rather rigid and ill-conceived boundary between public and private space. (Watson and Studdert 2006: 7)

Or at least they used to. Some, particularly those regarded as 'rougher round the edges', have been gradually wound down through a combination of rising rents and alleged mismanagement: seven of London's 90 or so street markets shut between 2008 and 2014 according to the Greater London Authority Conservatives' *Market Stalled* report (2013). Where they survive, one of the obvious consequences of the foodie boom is the disappearance of stalls selling more affordable fare, and their replacement with olive bars, smoked cheese vendors, and traders selling home-made cupcakes and artisanal breads:

> In the gentrified market, the focus is on specialty produce, particularly food (organic, hyper-local, artisanal), vintage clothes and independent fashion designers. The idea of a market as a gastronomic destination is emphasized. Essential goods such as affordable fresh fruit, vegetables, meat and fish become secondary or disappear, or for example rather than sell fresh fruit, stalls sell prepared trays with cut fruit at much higher prices. Customers also change. The market becomes a destination for higher-income shoppers looking for a special produce or tourists who are prepared to pay much higher prices. There's a sense of "distinction" of shopping at a market to differentiate oneself from the standardised supermarkets. (Gonzalez and Dawson 2015: 21)

In some cases, this upscaling has been an explicit part of urban regenerations agendas. For example, many boroughs have sought to use markets as strategic tools for regenerating place, with some—e.g. Broadway Market, Borough Market, Brixton Market, Chatsworth Road Market—appearing particularly important in pushing gentrification into once unfashionable neighbourhoods. Regan Koch and Alan Latham (2014: 151) conclude many markets now seem 'oriented toward attracting tourists or meeting the needs of the middle classes, rather than providing regular conveniences or amenities for a range of local residents'.

One of the most interesting trends here is the rise of the weekly High Street Farmers' Market. Typically held during a weekend, there were only a handful of these in Britain in the 1990s, with the first established in Bath in 1997. However, today they number, at a conservative estimate, around 550 (Spiller 2012). Some of these have been proclaimed as turning round the fortunes of traditional street markets, such as the new Broadway Food Market, which began in 2004 and now attracts 20,000 weekly according to its website. Running down from London Fields to the Regent's canal, this is a prime site of retail gentrification, with boutiques gradually replacing the locally oriented cafés and stores which front onto the weekly market boasting around 135 stalls. Like many other Farmers' Markets, Broadway does not actually involve many farmers selling to consumers, but there's an impressive range of artisanal and seasonal goods, along with stalls and trucks selling street foods including deep-fried arancini, Vietnamese pho rolls, organic feta filo pastries. Although the market's website suggests 90% of shoppers live locally, an independent (unpublished) survey carried out in 2004 suggested the average shopper had lived in the area for just nine months, going on to quote some longer-established Hackney residents who bemoaned the fact the market did not have the products they needed (see *Hackney Independent* 2004). Elsewhere, there's been criticism of the price of loaves of bread (typically £3–£5) unaffordable to a 'woman with three kids, a single parent' (Davies 2010: np).

While Hackney has been very much on the 'gentrification frontier' in the last decade, the idea that Farmers' Markets do not always serve the wider resident population can be evidenced elsewhere. Whitstable, for example, remains well-served by in-town supermarkets (a *Morrisons*, a *Co-op* and a *Budgens*) even though it has undergone dramatic foodie-led gentrification in the last decade. But wandering around its twice-monthly Farmers' Market it's hard to see who, apart from the more-affluent local residents and down-from-London weekenders might be able to afford Black Winter Truffle at £500 per kilo (Fig. 8.2), let alone the £4 artisanal breads, luxury ice creams, Godmersham-estate game pies and *Zinzie* hand-made cakes. All the stallholders come from within 30 miles of Whitstable, and enthusiastically extoll the virtues of local, organic and fair trade produce. One of the stallholders works out of an industrial unit not far from my own home, and he takes a good few minutes to explain the ethos of his business selling marinated olives. He tells me that his is one of the very few businesses in the country that chooses its olives before harvest, and imports the world's only fully traceable PDO (Protected Designation of Origin) olive oil, whose precise source he is able to track via GPS down to specific hillsides in Crete. He encourages me to take a swig of extra virgin, and appreciate its peppery notes. As the buttery foretaste gives way to intense heat, I feel vaguely nauseous and I am not in any way keen to purchase, but I do not show any displeasure lest I offend

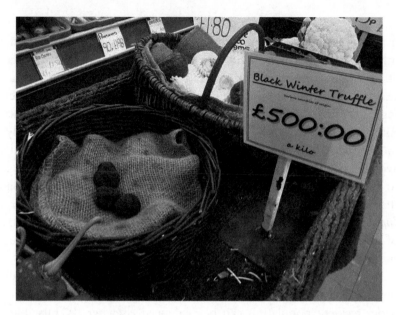

Fig. 8.2 Produce at Whitstable farmer's market (photo: Katie Blythe, used with permission)

him. Indeed, like a lot of people there I am not actually buying much, but I am wallowing in the generally feel-good atmosphere, reveling in an opportunity to display my cultural capital to others.

So, although Farmers' Markets have been important in reconnecting consumers to the social, cultural and environmental contexts of food production (Smith et al. 2014), and appear to be encouraging a general emphasis on food quality over food quantity, there's now an international academic literature confirming they mainly serve the appetites of middle-class consumers. Leslie Kern (2015a), for example, charts the gentrification of the Junction district in Toronto—once notorious for street sex work, drug dealing, 'toxicity', industry, litter and meatpacking—suggesting the Farmers' Market helped re-narrate the neighbourhood as eco-conscious, an area typified by a 'crunchy chic'. The organic and healthy goods sold at the market were taken as symbolic of the transformation of the area, from masculine to feminine, toxic to clean, contaminated to pure. As she details, numerous cafés 'specializing in local and organic meals and coffee as well as vegetarian and vegan options, organic groceries, gluten-free bakeries, natural pet product stores, artisan meat and cheese shops, fitness centres, and yoga and Pilates studios' also sprung up, directly displaced other businesses, 'including greasy spoon diners, porn shops, and dollar stores' (Kern 2015a: 75). While this was a clear case of retail gentrification, Kern suggests this was sublimated into a language in which the 'turf war' between middle-class and working-class residents was cast as a battle between different land uses: sex shops versus vegan restaurants, dirty diners versus cafés selling wholesome wholefoods. While Rachel Slocum (2007: 7) is less concerned with gentrification per se, her research notes Farmers' Markets can be involved in the maintenance of a distinctly white, middle-class sense of community, suggesting these are spaces where 'whites come together, stick together and become impenetrable to Others despite the desire to be otherwise'. It can also be a space where certain foodstuffs are depicted as local and authentic, and hence implied to be healthy when they are often nothing of the sort (e.g. 'traditional' artisanal ice cream, pulled pork burgers and regional cheeses are indulgent, high-fat foods). The conflation of health, wholesomeness and localness in these spaces is then potentially problematic, and not only in instances where stallholders or growers are uniformly white and middle class: sometimes the consumption of 'non-white food' in such spaces provides a means by which white middle-class professionals can exhibit their distinction and cosmopolitan superiority (see Guthman 2008, on Latino traders at US Farmers' Markets).

British Farmers' Markets are not immune from such critiques. Sara Gonzalez and Paul Waley maintain street markets in Britain remain 'among the public spaces where migrant communities are most visible', but suggest they risk 'the potential consumerist commodification of the ethnic other' with 'ethnic' food, fabrics, or arts and crafts stalls 'spicing up' the market experience for 'food adventurers':

Paraphrasing [Neil] Smith's analysis of the frontier myth in New York, one could envisage "pioneers" discovering the "quirky" side of markets, venturing into this space, and enjoying the "mixing" and the rubbing-along effect. These pioneers like the feeling of being in a different space not yet colonised by corporate values; they enjoy the fact that they have "discovered" a place that is still not frequented by people like them (i.e. middle and upper classes). (Gonzalez and Waley 2012: 971)

The argument here is urgent and compelling and suggests the Farmers' Market is a space associated with an incipient gentrification that can gradually alienate poorer and non-white residents. Indeed, Gonzalez and Waley's (2012) focus on the gentrification of the covered markets of Leeds under-scores many of the points made in this section about the potential dangers of a High Street regeneration which particularly values the taste cultures associated with 'foodism'. In a society where cultural capital is displayed by showing an appreciation of the quality and provenance of food, and particularly 'slow' foods, working-class food practices are marginalized and access to affordable staple foodstuffs given a low priority. Given the now-record numbers using food banks in the UK (over a million receiving three-days' emergency food supply from Trussell Trust food banks in 2015), this is serious cause for concern.

Obesogenic Urbanism and 'Climate Friendly' Food

The gentrification of urban foodscapes raises serious questions about fairness and equity in society, with attempts at upscaling the High Street food offer being broadly welcomed despite the obvious impacts this might have in terms of limiting the choices for those who cannot afford artisanal loaves and traceable olive oils. After all, it's difficult to argue against food depicted as green, healthy and environmentally sustainable, particularly when it emerges on High Streets otherwise dominated by fast food outlets, which 69% think, discourage healthy choices, and 50% think, cause mental health problems (Royal Society of Public Health 2015). As we have seen, the High Street is believed to play the most significant role in what has become known as the UK's 'obesity epidemic' (Morland and Evenson 2009). While few suggest the High Street is inherently obesogenic (as the relation between obesity and the types of food offered in different environments is shaped by personal taste as well as intervening factors like exercise or energy expenditure), there's a body of opinion suggesting that relatively minor changes to the High Street might successfully mediate these relations to produce healthier outcomes. Paramount here is the aforementioned planning crackdown on the fast food takeaways serving energy-dense, calorific meals that can be consumed on the street, often in large portions. These outlets are indelibly associated with a discredited working class variously portrayed as lazy and unhealthy, with images of obesity prevalent in media coverage of their impact on community well-being (Graham-Leigh 2015).

Describing people as overweight can, if one draws on Michel Foucault's ideas, be seen as a form of neoliberal governmentality that invents particular 'norms' by drawing attention to extreme cases (e.g. the obese or the bulimic). The discursive chaining of fatness to unhealthiness is significant in this respect given this is a conflation which encourages particular forms of 'care for the self', including the consumption of particular 'healthy' foods which are often more expensive than 'unhealthy' alternatives. In a situation where 65% of men and 56% of women are currently classified as overweight in England (HSCIC 2014), and one-third of all adults described as 'clinically' obese, the policy fixation with limiting the availability of fast food on the High Street is explicable both as an attempt to valorize these more expensive options as well as condemning cheaper food consumption as a sign of poor self-control or lack of education. Kebabs, fish and chips, pasties, burgers, deep-fried chicken and pizzas all offer affordable, hot, filling food for those on the go, but it's often assumed in the media it's the 'obese' who frequent such outlets, while those who have thin, toned, bodies are thought to exhibit forms of restraint and self-control which mean they shun them. Such assumptions are, of course, potentially misleading, as bodies can never reveal the true effort involved in their own making (Guthman 2009). Diet is clearly only part of the story when it comes to body size.

Irrespective of the tenuous relationship of eating and body size, patronage of takeaway food outlets is frequently linked to low diet quality and weight gain. For example, in a study published in the *British Medical Journal*, Tim Burgoine et al. (2014) reviewed longitudinal health data relating to the eating habits and Body Mass Index of some 5500 individuals, and concluded that the group most exposed to takeaway food outlets had a significantly higher Body Mass Index than those less exposed. This group was also 38% more likely to be obese than those least exposed. In the same study, researchers estimated grams of daily takeaway consumption based on intake of burgers, pizza, fried chicken and chips. The group of people who were most exposed to fast food options consumed on average 39.9 g grams per week more takeaway food than the least exposed group, a small but apparently significant amount (equivalent to around half a serving of *McDonalds* French fries).

But it's important to remember the High Street is not the only place where fast food and unhealthy options are encountered, as many people are offered, and consume, fast food at home, at school and in the workplace too: it's estimated the average person encounters 32 different takeaway options on a daily basis (Burgoine et al. 2014). It's also important to bear in mind that it's not just deep-fried food that is highly calorific, as some 'healthy' options (including pre-packaged salads and sandwiches) contain more fat than the average burger and fries, meaning a *Pret a Manger, Marks and Spencer* or *Waitrose* could be just as damaging to public health as a chicken shop. Ecological studies nonetheless suggest there are typically more fast food and takeaway outlets in those areas with higher rates of obesity. But even here we need to be careful in drawing spurious causation from correlation, as the association of obesity and the presence of fast food outlets may be an example of the 'deprivation amplification' effect given residents in deprived areas have poorer access to health-promoting resources (e.g. health clubs, gyms, open spaces, doctors' surgeries) than residents in more-affluent areas (Fraser et al. 2010). Combined with studies arguing the presence of fast food restaurants alone is not a contextual driver of health-based inequalities (e.g. Pearce et al. 2009), and proximity to fast food restaurants is not a good predictor of whether one is actually likely to eat in them (e.g. Jeffrey et al. 2006), it appears deprivation is more associated with obesity than the presence of fast food takeaways per se. Overall, the inability of working-class populations to afford active lifestyles or buy healthier low-fat, low-salt foods is probably a more significant factor encouraging obesity than the presence of fast food takeaways in the local 'food environment'.

Despite this ambivalent evidence, policies promoting healthier diets continue to argue that reducing neighbourhood exposure to takeaway food is important. However, the fight to remove fast food from our High Street also deploys other arguments, as Elaine Graham-Leigh (2015) shows when she highlights the importance of so-called *climate-friendly food*. As she explains, the suggestion that those consuming nutrient-poor, energy-dense food in the urban West are responsible both for climate change and a global shortage of food is now a widely accepted argument. Rather than blaming global inequality for such issues, it's the consumption habits of the 'obese' that is highlighted. But not all of those who are obese appear equally to blame: news stories about obesity are not routinely illustrated with images of fat people in business suits tucking into expensive steaks in upscale restaurants. Instead, we see images of 'headless fatties' in jogging pants tucking into burgers in the street, apparently feckless and thoughtless in their consumption practices. The logic becomes clear: the poor are over-consuming, encouraging the fast food chains to produce beef as cheaply as possible, exacerbating the environmental and social costs of production (e.g. increased methane emissions, costs of transportation, deforestation to make way for pasture). The answer? Shut down the fast food restaurants that offer cheap beef in an effort to reduce both obesity and climate change. All good, but why is cheap beef seen to be 'bad food' while more expensive beef is fine? It's a question worth asking at a time when the fashion for expensive gourmet burgers continues apace: why is it fine for people to be able to buy a 'proper' burger at *Byron Burgers* for £6.95 (a 6 oz hamburger in a bun) whereas a cheaper alternative—e.g. a 1.3 oz *McDonalds* burger for 99p—is apparently responsible for reckless overproduction and the obesity epidemic?

The labeling of certain forms of consumption as damaging to the environment is then part of a wider moralizing narrative which depicts the consumption choices of the working classes as excessive, selfish and unhealthy. In truth, neither *McDonalds*, obese people or 'toxic' British High Streets should have to bear the brunt of responsibility for a capitalist system that has encouraged contemporary modes of food production and consumption. But no matter, as policies designed to push cheap burger joints and fast food takeaways off, our High Streets are now being spread as a matter of best practice. Whether these will have any of the intended effects in terms of improving obesity rates, or reducing littering and noise, remains to be seen, although evidence from other contexts suggest that this is something of a forlorn hope. Indeed, in reviewing the effects of a ban on new fast food outlets in South Central Los Angeles, Roland Sturm and Aiko Hattori (2015) conclude that, five years on, this had little demonstrable effect. Indeed, their research questions the initial logic of a ban in this part of LA, suggesting fruit and vegetable consumption in this area was never out of kilter with other areas of the city, and arguing that the increase in obesity and fast food consumption in this area was also in line with neighbouring areas. Viewed in this light, the targeting of an area with a significant African-American and Latino majority appears to be an example of environmental racism, with state policies imposing particular behavioural norms on minority populations on the basis they are particularly prevalent to food-related mortality and morbidity. In the process, their relative deprivation is elided, and their poor diet seen to be the outcome of poor individual choices and lack of restraint rather than lack of money.

Despite this, British local authorities continue to move forward with policies designed to make it harder to open hot food takeaways. Interestingly, of the 20 or so local authorities who had introduced controls by 2015, the majority were urban areas typified by both higher than average deprivation and non-white occupation: Newham, Tower Hamlets, Sandwell, Stoke, Barking & Dagenham, Medway, Birmingham, and Plymouth amongst others. In some areas, like the Mile End road in Tower Hamlets (which has around 43 chicken shops by some estimates) it might be said that this type of restrictive policy is long overdue. After all, on top of the arguments about obesity, climate change and unsustainable consumption practices, we have seen that some middle-class consumers proclaim them as eyesores on the 'traditional' British High Street. There's little counter-discourse here, or any sense that this blanket condemnation needs to be tempered with a more nuanced appreciation of the role they play in the lives of many poorer populations, particularly younger people growing up in environments where there are few other spaces in which to socialize. A rare exception is Townshend's (2016: 16) study of the local shopping streets in Newcastle riddled with fast food takeaways. In this, he draws on interviews and focus groups to suggest the presence of food outlets 'might be viewed as not wholly negative since they add life and use to areas that might otherwise be largely lifeless' noting 'some provide foci for some minority groups, both as an economic opportunity and as a meeting venue'. He continues by suggesting that minority ethnic groups, urban designers and planners might 'productively explore whether those positives of vitality and providing space for social interaction' might be harnessed to promote healthier lifestyles.

Ironically, one of the only other defenses mounted of the chicken shop takeaway has been by arch-foodie Jay Rayner, *The Observer's* restaurant critic. He argues:

> For school-age children the fried-chicken shops are now "third spaces" between the classroom and home. For certain urban tribes they're like train stations: a fixed point through which life crosses back and forth. In the way of cities not all of it is shiny and positive; they have been associated with gang crime and antisocial behaviour. Bad things sometimes happen in them, and around them, which has nothing to do with dismal food. At other times, however, they operate more as refuge than food dispensary. (Rayner 2013: np)

This is hardly unqualified support for chicken shops, but the notion they provide refuges in the modern city resonates well with my own observations. For example, when working with a group of young, unaccompanied asylum seekers in a project focusing on their experience of moving to the East Midlands (O'Neill and Hubbard 2010), it was usual for us to meet up in the local chicken shop before we went on to the local venue where we rehearsed a play telling their stories of relocation. Mainly 16 or 17, these young men were mainly Iraqi Kurds, Afghanis or Bosnians, studying at the local college, and living in shared houses lacking much in the way of space to hang out. The chicken shop where one of their friends worked became their key meeting point, a place where they could sit and chat without experiencing the hassle they sometimes got from local white kids in the town park, or when playing football at the recreation ground. The proprietor seemed happy to accommodate them, allowing them to charge their phones in his sockets even if they were often not consuming anything more than a can of fizzy drink (50p). But once a week, they got a payment courtesy of the National Asylum Support Service of £17. Routinely, when it arrived, they would spend £4 or £5 straight away at the chicken shop on a large meal of six fried halal chicken wings, large fries, a tub of coleslaw, and a bottle of coke, sharing it with friends who lacked even that meager level of financial support.

This type of sociality and generosity may not be typical of all chicken shops. However, Shift's (2012) observational study suggests around half of those visiting chicken shops are under 18, with around 20% of them ordering nothing, implying they are significant as a meeting space, and not just as an eating place. And while half of those visiting chicken shops leave within four minutes of them or their friends receiving their food, around a third are still there 20 minutes later. So even though one suspects few will mourn the gradual disappearance of *Tennessee Fried Chicken*, *Dixie Chicken*, *Fat Sam's* or *Euro Fried Chicken* from British High Streets, if they are not replaced by shops selling equally affordable fare, the outcome will be a form of retail gentrification that may have particular consequences for less-affluent, non-white consumers, mirroring the type of shifts occurring in many gentrifying North American neighbourhoods: a shift from fast food to slow food, and from outlets where the poorer feel comfortable to ones where they palpably do not. As Karen Franck (2005: 6) argues, we need to marry the 'culinary evidence of urban regeneration and gentrification with contradictory feelings of pleasure and dismay': pleasure in the fact that our cities offer more luxurious, potentially healthier and wider food choices than ever before, but dismay that some of the well-loved, well-used eateries frequented by working class and ethnic minority consumers are now beleaguered spaces being sacrificed in the name of regeneration.

References

Augé, M. (1995). *Non-place*. London: Verso.

Bell, D., & Hollows, J. (2011). From River Cottage to Chicken Run: Hugh Fearnley-Whittingstall and the class politics of ethical consumption. *Celebrity Studies, 2*(2), 178–191.

Blythman, J. (2010). *Bad food Britain: How a nation ruined its appetite*. London: Fourth Estate.

Browning, B. (2014). Costa coffee announces plans for new store in the market place, Faversham. *Kent Online*, 13 May, http://www.kentonline.co.uk/faversham/news/costa-set-to-take-on-17165/

Burgoine, T., Forouhi, N. G., Griffin, S. J., Wareham, N. J., & Monsivais, P. (2014). Associations between exposure to takeaway food outlets, takeaway food consumption, and body weight in Cambridgeshire, UK: A population based, cross-sectional study. *British Medical Journal, 348*, g1464.

Caraher, M., O'Keefe, E., Lloyd, S., & Madelin, T. (2013). The planning system and fast food outlets in London: Lessons for health promotion practice. *Revista Portuguesa de Saúde Pública, 31*(1), 49–57.

Carpenter, J. (2012). Councils call for powers to halt betting shop clustering, Planning Resource, 28 February, http://www.planningresource.co.uk/article/1119449/councils-call-powers-halt-betting-shop-clustering

Colls, R. (2007). Materialising bodily matter: Intra-action and the embodiment of 'fat'. *Geoforum, 38*(2), 353–365.

Cookney, R. (2014). Fast food mile: The school run that has 34 takeaways on one road. *The Daily Mirror*, 26 April, http://www.mirror.co.uk/news/uk-news/fast-food-mile-school-run-3463153

Crewe, L. (2008). Ugly beautiful? Counting the cost of the global fashion industry. *Geography, 93*(1), 25.

Crewe, L. (2016). *Geographies of fashion: Consumption, space and value*. London: Bloomsbury.

Davies, A. (2010). Broadway goes upmarket. *Hackney Citizen*, 12 February. http://hackneycitizen.co.uk/2010/02/12/hackney-goes-up-market/

Department for Environment, Food and Rural Affairs (2004). *Reducing litter caused by food on the go': A voluntary code of practice for local partnerships*. London: Defra.

Department of Health (2008). *Healthy weight, healthy lives*. London: HMSO.

Elias, N. (1982). *The civilizing process*. New York: Pantheon Books.

Evans, B., & Colls, R. (2009). Measuring fatness, governing bodies: The spatialities of the Body Mass Index (BMI) in anti-obesity politics. *Antipode, 41*(5), 1051–1083.

Everts, J., & Jackson, P. (2009). Modernisation and the practices of contemporary food shopping. *Environment and Planning D: Society and Space, 27*(5), 917–935.

Franck, K. A. (2005). The city as dining room, market and farm. *Architectural Design, 75*(3), 5–10.

Fraser, L. K., Edwards, K. L., Cade, J., & Clarke, G. P. (2010). The geography of fast food outlets: A review. *International Journal of Environmental Research and Public Health, 7*(5), 2290–2308.

Gentleman, A. (2012). Cheap meat and exploitation behind the chicken shop counter. *The Guardian*, 29 June, http://www.theguardian.com/business/2012/jun/29/chicken-shop-raids

Gonzalez, S. and Dawson, G. (2015). Traditional markets under threat: Why it's happening and what traders and customers can do. http://tradmarketresearch.weebly.com/uploads/4/5/6/7/45677825/traditional_markets_under_threat-_full.pdf

Gonzalez, S., & Waley, P. (2012). Traditional retail markets: The new gentrification frontier? *Antipode, 45*(4), 965–983.

Graham-Leigh, E. (2015). *A diet of austerity: Class, food and climate change.* London: Zero Books.

Greater London Authority (2012). *Takeaways toolkit.* London: GLA.

Greater London Authority (2013). *Open for business: Empty shops on London's High Streets.* London: GLA.

Gregson, N., Crewe, L., & Brooks, K. (2002). Shopping, space, and practice. *Environment and Planning (D)—Society and Space, 20*(5), 597–618.

Guthman, J. (2008). "If they only knew": Color blindness and universalism in California alternative food institutions. *The Professional Geographer, 60*(3), 387–397.

Guthman, J. (2009). Teaching the politics of obesity: Insights into neoliberal embodiment and contemporary biopolitics. *Antipode, 41*(5), 1110–1133.

Hackney Independent. (2004). A market for Hackney's new yuppies. Hackney Independent, Haggerston edition, Winter 2004, http://www.hackneyindependent.org/wp-content/uploads/2011/08/win04.pdf

Hall, S. M. (2011). High Street adaptations: Ethnicity, independent retail practices, and localism in London's urban margins. *Environment and Planning A, 43*(11), 2571–2588.

Hattersley, G. (2006). We know what food kids like best, and it's not polenta. *The Sunday Times* 24 September, 14.

Health & Social Care Information Centre (2014). *Statistics on obesity, physical activity and diet, England.* London: HSCIC.

Highmore, B. (2008). Alimentary agents: Food, cultural theory and multiculturalism. *Journal of Intercultural studies, 29*(4), 381–398.

Hoskins, T. E. (2014). *Stitched up: The anti-capitalist book of fashion.* London: Pluto Press.

Hughes, D. (1995). Animal welfare: The consumer and the food industry. *British Food Journal, 97*(10), 3–7.

Jabs, J., & Devine, C. M. (2006). Time scarcity and food choices: An overview. *Appetite, 47*(2), 196–204.

Jackson, P. (2016). Go Home Jamie: Reframing consumer choice. *Social & Cultural Geography.* doi:10.1080/14649365.2015.1124912.

Jackson, P., & Viehoff, V. (2016). Reframing convenience food. *Appetite, 98*, 1–11.

Jeffery, R. W., Baxter, J., McGuire, M., & Linde, J. (2006). Are fast food restaurants an environmental risk factor for obesity? *International Journal of Behavioral Nutrition & Physical Activity, 3*(1), 1–12.

Kern, L. (2015a). From toxic wreck to crunchy chic: Environmental gentrification through the body. *Environment and Planning D: Society and Space, 33,* 67–83.

Knox, P. L. (2005). Creating ordinary places: Slow cities in a fast world. *Journal of Urban Design, 10*(1), 1–11.

Koch, R., & Latham, A. (2014). Inhabiting cities, domesticating public space: Making sense of the changing public life of contemporary London. In A. Madanipour, S. Knierbein, & A. Degros (Eds.), *Public space and the challenges of transformation in Europe.* London: Routledge.

Maguire, E. R., Burgoine, T., & Monsivais, P. (2015). Area deprivation and the food environment over time: A repeated cross-sectional study on takeaway outlet density and supermarket presence in Norfolk, UK, 1990–2008. *Health & Place, 33,* 142–147.

Marshall, D. (2005). Food as ritual, routine or convention. *Consumption Markets & Culture, 8*(1), 69–85.

McDonalds and Allegra Strategies (2009). *Eating out in the UK 2009: A comprehensive analysis of the informal eating out market.* London: Allegra.

McMichael, A. J., Powles, J. W., Butler, C. D., & Uauy, R. (2007). Food, livestock production, energy, climate change, and health. *The Lancet, 370*(9594), 1253–1263.

Merrifield, A. (2006). *Henri Lefebvre: A critical introduction.* London: Taylor & Francis.

Morland, K. B., & Evenson, K. R. (2009). Obesity prevalence and the local food environment. *Health & Place, 15*(2), 491–495.

New Economics Foundation (2003). *Ghost town Britain: The threat from economic globalisation to livelihoods, liberty and local freedom.* London: NEF.

New Economics Foundation (2010). *Re-imagining the High Street: Escape from clone town Britain.* London: NEF.

O'Neill, M., & Hubbard, P. (2010). Walking, sensing, belonging: Ethnomimesis as performative praxis. *Visual Studies, 25*(1), 46–58.

Pearce, J., Hiscock, R., Blakely, T., & Witten, K. (2009). A national study of the association between neighborhood access to fast-food outlets and the diet and weight of local residents. *Health & Place, 15*(1), 193–197.

Pike, J., & Leahy, D. (2012). School food and the pedagogies of parenting. *Australian Journal of Adult Learning, 52*(3), 434.

Potter, L., & Westall, C. (2013). Neoliberal Britain's austerity foodscape: Home economics, veg patch capitalism and culinary temporality. *New Formations: A Journal of Culture/Theory/Politics, 80*(80), 155–178.

Public Health England (2014). *Obesity and the environment: Regulating the growth of fast food outlets.* London: Public Health England.

Raynor, J. (2013). Fried chicken fix: After-school fast food. *The Guardian*, 26 October, http://www.theguardian.com/lifeandstyle/2013/oct/26/fried-chicken-fast food-shop-schoolkids

Rhys-Taylor, A. (2013). Disgust and distinction: The case of the jellied eel. *The Sociological Review*, 61(2), 227–246.

Rich, E. (2011). 'I see her being obesed!': Public pedagogy, reality media and the obesity crisis. *Health*, 15(1), 3–21.

Ritzer, G. (2003). Islands of the living dead the social geography of McDonaldization. *American Behavioral Scientist*, 47(2), 119–136.

Royal Society of Public Health (2015). *Health on the High Street*. London: RSPH.

Shift (2012). *Chicken shops and poor diet: Summary of research findings*. London: Shift.

Slocum, R. (2007). Whiteness, space and alternative food practice. *Geoforum*, 38(3), 520–533.

Smith, J., Maye, D., & Ilbery, B. (2014). The traditional food market and place: New insights into fresh food provisioning in England. *Area*, 46(1), 122–128.

Spiller, K. (2012). It tastes better because … consumer understandings of UK farmers' market food. *Appetite*, 59(1), 100–107.

Sturm, R., & Hattori, A. (2015). Diet and obesity in Los Angeles county 2007–2012: Is there a measurable effect of the 2008 "fast-food ban"? *Social Science & Medicine*, 133, 205–211.

Thompson, J. (2009). Britain's growing appetite for fast food is proving insatiable. The Independent, 25 November, http://www.independent.co.uk/news/business/analysis-and-features/britains-appetite-for-fast-food-is-proving-insatiable-1826902.html

Tokatli, N. (2008). Global sourcing: Insights from the global clothing industry—The case of Zara, a fast fashion retailer. *Journal of Economic Geography*, 8(1), 21–38.

Townshend, T. G. (2016). Toxic High Streets. *Journal of Urban Design*, online early, doi:10.1080/13574809.2015.1106916

Valentine, G. (1998). Food and the production of the civilised street. In N. Fyfe (Ed.), *Images of the street: Planning identity and control in public space*. London: Routledge.

Watson, S., & Studdert, D. (2006). *Markets as sites for social interaction: Spaces of diversity*. Bristol: Policy Press.

9

Bohemia on the High Street

So far, we have seen that in the battle to revive the fortunes of the High Street, particular businesses are valued over others. Slow food trumps fast food, and takeaways condemned. A high-class sex emporium might be okay, but 'old-fashioned' sex shops and lap dance clubs certainly are not. Betting shops are bad, as are discount pubs and off-licenses promoting cheap alcohol. Given all these businesses are capable of maintaining footfall and attracting customers to the High Street, it isn't clear that the distinctions drawn between toxic and virtuous businesses are about the vitality and viability of local shopping streets. Rather, there seems to be a conscious attempt to re-moralize the High Street via a deliberative policy push favouring particular forms of consumption over others. Within such visions, the working class are abject (Haylett 2001). Their lifestyles, tastes and needs are barely registered. In a sense, their views do not even matter. For in the contemporary context of 'austerity urbanism' (Peck 2012), local authorities appear to have given up on the idea they might invest in the needs of working-class communities and those on benefits. Instead, they act in entrepreneurial ways, seeking to lever in investment from the private sector. This is, of course, easiest in the context of housing, with 'seriously under-valued' council housing estates being developed into

© The Editor(s) (if applicable) and The Author(s) 2017   **199**
P. Hubbard, *The Battle for the High Street*,
DOI 10.1057/978-1-137-52153-8_9

'mixed housing' by corporations encouraged to do this by local authorities who lack the imagination or willingness to explore other models of regeneration. But it's also something closely associated with attempts to regenerate High Streets. In effect, many of our town and city centres are being remade in the image of the corporations' target market: hip, young, affluent populations who are prepared to pay a premium for city living, and expect the High Street to match their gentrified lifestyles.

The suggestion here is that retail gentrification can be a state-sponsored phenomenon, with local authorities keen to knock the awkward edges off the High Street, sacrificing those businesses that do not quite fit the image of a prosperous twenty-first-century city. Apparently, they'd rather have a vacant shop rather than one that creates the 'wrong impression', except that they would never say that—at least not in so many words. Rather than being upfront about their intentions, this desire to cleanse the city of its gritty working-class heritage is expressed in a more neutral language. Policies advocating retail regeneration are framed in terms of improving general amenity, creating more attractive, inclusive and livable High Streets. The rhetoric consequently gives considerable weight to the value of the 'local' and the 'independent', as opposed to the 'inauthenticity' associated with retail multiples. Notions of 'resilience' also get a look-in here, with the idea that businesses like betting shops, discount stores and takeaways add little to the long-term sustainability of a local shopping street often stressed. But no less significant is the idea that cities need to be *creative* to compete in the contemporary global economy. Consequently, many declining High Streets are being re-imagined as spaces that might incubate and foster a wider creative transformation in Britain. For example, in 2015 the Mayor of London's High Street Fund pledged up to £20,000 to 17 community projects as part of an ongoing attempt to support regeneration, with over a third of these supporting cultural and creative projects including a roving pop-up comedy shop in vacant units on Romford High Street, a new cultural quarter in Roehampton and artists' workspaces in Haringey. Equally, many Portas pilot towns have explored ways of developing creativity on the High Street (e.g. Brighton's London Road markets itself as a 'social conscience, community, affordable, creative industry cluster', Bedminster has tried to build on Bristol's reputation for street art by providing subsidized workshop spaces in disused shops, and Loughborough's 'Market Town' project has witnessed schoolchildren taking over abandoned shops and filling them with their art, overseen by local artists). Of course, there's a degree of expediency here, as during the retail recession 'creatives' provide landlord-friendly ways to occupy the growing 'slack space' on High Streets as market demand falls, providing a cheap anti-squatting security service for landlords as well providing a source of rent. But such activity is by no means limited to the UK. For example, Katharine Rankin and Heather McLean (2015) write from a North American perspective suggesting that in planning and policy circles, the promotion of vibrant, artful shopping streets has become a basic staple of 'creative city planning', with similar tendencies noted in places as diverse as Singapore (Chang 2016), New Zealand (Latham 2003) and Chile (Schlack and Turnbull 2015).

The creative city idea—encapsulated in the policy toolkit offered by Charles Landry and Franco Bianchini (1995), and theoretically buttressed through the ideas of Richard Florida (2002)—has become globally hegemonic in urban policy. This essentially revolves the idea that declining cities—and failing shopping streets within these—can be revivified through the production of a creative vibe which will appeal to artists and allied members of the 'creative class'. Though the exact nature of this creative vibe remains elusive, in this chapter I want to suggest that the distinction often made between the 'creative' and 'uncreative' classes threatens to inform the production of 'artful' spaces that can knowingly exclude established working-class residents. Perhaps the most obvious example of this 'artwashing' is provided by the colonization of the East End of London by artists and creatives over the last couple of decades. However, after exploring the hipster invasion of Hoxton and Shoreditch, I'll return to Margate, where culture-led regeneration has been held up as a panacea to the problems associated with a declining town centre. Through these case studies, I want to question whether creative policies can succeed in broadening the appeal of the High Street, or will merely precipitate the 'boutiqueing' and gentrification of retail space.

Culture-Led Urban Regeneration

In post-industrial societies, where manufacturing has grudgingly given way to a new 'weightless' economy, knowledge and creativity are frequently described as the raw materials of economic prosperity. Given this emphasis, it's widely believed that the creative industries are major drivers of wealth and job creation, tied into the emergence of forms of consumption which are fast-moving, highly segmented and increasingly cultural (O'Connor 2000). But more than this, creativity is encouraged as it's seen as a way of promoting cultural diversity, being theoretically able to nurture local distinctiveness and difference (Pratt 2011). Consequently, under New Labour in particular, many reports on national competitiveness suggested that the creative industries represented a panacea for decline and disinvestment. For example, the 2001 Creative Industries Task Force defined the creative industries as 'those industries which have their origin in individual creativity, skill and talent and which have a potential for wealth and job creation through the generation and exploitation of intellectual property', estimating this sector contributed 8% of gross domestic product, and was expanding at a rate of around 9% per annum (compared with 2.8% growth in the entire UK economy) (DCMS 2001).

The identification of the creative industries as a driver of the national economy means creativity has been a potent symbolic territory in the twenty-first-century city (Jayne 2005; Peck 2005). In Britain, this has been mirrored in a gamut of attempts to foster innovation and creativity through the designation of post-industrial cultural or creative quarters. The development of the Gateshead Quayside in Newcastle, focused on the construction of the Millennium Bridge, the conversion of the Baltic Flour Mill into an art gallery, and the building of the Sage, a music and arts centre, at a cost of £22 million, £45 million and £70 million respectively, provides a particularly prominent example. Others include Sheffield's Cultural Industries Quarter, Stoke's Cultural Quarter and Birmingham's Creative Quarter, the latter based around the former Bird's custard factory which provides workspaces for musicians, digital artists and graphic designers. But it's not only the larger cities that have sought to boost their creative industries, with smaller cities and towns (e.g. Wakefield, Huddersfield and Folkestone) having developed designated cultural districts. In each case, the hope is to create a vibrant and innovative milieu in which creative industries can flourish.

In many of these cases, culture-led regeneration has become synonymous with arts-led regeneration. The infamous English transvestite ceramicist Grayson Perry suggests as much when he argues artists are at the vanguard of processes that symbolically embellish and unlock the potential of place:

> The currency of bohemian-ness, lefty, arty-fartiness ... has a high currency, especially in the urban ecology. And if you think of artists, they're like the shock troops of gentrification. We march in. We're the first people to go "We like this old warehouse, yeah we need a cheap studio". You know so that's what happens—artists move into the cheap housing and the cheap spaces ... they do their work and they're quite cool and a little bit of a buzz starts up. And then maybe a little café opens up and people start saying, "Ooh, that's kind of interesting, that area where those artists hang out. I think I'm going to go down there"... And people start noticing, you know, and maybe some designers open up a little boutique ... And before you know it, the developers move in and that's it—bang goes the area. (Perry 2013: 7)

The presence of artists—particularly visual artists—is understood to be 'a catalyst for neighbourhood transition' (Bridge 2006: 1965), converting 'urban dilapidation into ultra chic' (Smith 1996: 18). Here, both the visible presence of the arts (e.g. in terms of the emergence of gallery and workshop spaces) and the reputational change associated with this (e.g. the caché attached to artistic lifestyles) transforms the symbolic meaning of urban spaces and stimulates economic development (Mathews 2014). The construction of a flagship art gallery or exhibition space is assumed by many local authorities to be the way of kick-starting this process. The Public in West Bromwich, the New Art Gallery, Walsall, Mima in Middlesborough, the Hepworth in Wakefield, the Jerwood in Hastings, the Turner in Margate, and Colchester's Firstsite all follow the formula: architect-designed spaces intended to transform dreary provincialism into edgy, cultural cool. As Stuart Cameron and Jon Coaffee (2005: 54) argue, such galleries demonstrate 'the potential power of an arts- and culture-based regeneration strategy to give rise to gentrification in the most unlikely of locations' (see also Harvie 2013). The recipe here is a well-tested import:

Sharon Zukin (1995: 21) notes that, in the USA, almost every downtown has an artists' quarter, with disused factories or waterfront sites converted into a 'sites of visual delectation—a themed shopping space for seasonal produce, cooking equipment, restaurants, art galleries'. The same is now true in Britain, with the new generation of subsidized galleries anchoring a mix of cool consumption spaces that it's hoped will attract visitors to what are otherwise uncelebrated towns.

The cultivation of an artful image and ambience has hence become *de rigeur* in recessionary times, and one well matched to areas with derelict and vacant properties given low-rent units have appeal to artists. But there's a wider logic to these approaches, as arts-based identities can be easily marshalled in place marketing efforts drawing attention to 'authentic' local character and heritage. Such 'cultural hard branding approaches' may be serially replicated, but still seem vital in attracting new forms of investor and investment in global times. Here, the work of Richard Florida (2002) remains influential, his idea that quality of life and cultural liberalism attract the 'creative class' a significant influence on creative city policy. In his view, regions and cities develop competitive advantage based on their ability to create new business ideas and commercial products. Such innovation, he argues, depends on the concentration of highly educated, knowledge-rich and inevitably mobile workers within a given locale. These are the creative workers who, Florida alleges, give city economies their cutting edge, and allow certain cities to out-perform their rivals. While Florida's (2002) analysis stresses the importance of creative individuals in a wide variety of fields—engineering, design, management—his ideas are highly relevant to explaining why some cities are promoting arts-led regeneration. In effect, he argues that the key to competitive advantage is the ability of a city to attract and retain creative individuals by emphasizing their cultural credentials (Peck 2005). Given that Florida asserts that creative people shun the suburbs in favour of 'happening' and tolerant inner city districts, he suggests this may involve the conscious marketing and commodification of urban quarters that boast amenities including restaurants, coffee shops, wine bars, music venues and galleries. For Florida (2002) these facilities, where consumption, networking, and 'experiences' can occur, provide the necessary ambience necessary to attract the 'creative class'.

A much-cited example of cultural regeneration in action is the Wicker Park district of Chicago, a formerly industrial, partly derelict and largely Latino inner city neighbourhood that was seized upon by the US media in the 1990s as a 'cutting-edge' district of street-level music and art production, consequently becoming a magnet for artists, students and young professionals. In this case, the ethnic diversity, grit and cosmopolitanism of the area appeared a major lure for artists who, inevitably, reduced the heterogeneity of the area (the majority being white and middle class). Richard Lloyd (2002) concludes that some of the characteristics perceived by urban politicians as liabilities can be important in fostering culturally led growth. Before long, vacant and derelict properties along the main strip of Milwaukee Avenue were opened as bars, art galleries and funky shops. Visiting in 2006, I was surprised at the sheer number of shabby chic coffee shops packed with Mac-wielding creative types who spilled onto the pavement, mingling with tattooed cyclists. Admittedly, the street was still home to a good number of longer-established thrift stores and 'ethnic' restaurants, but these were outnumbered by vintage furniture stores, gourmet sandwich shops and tastefully renovated bars serving local microbrews. I even noted a hipster infant-wear store selling punk-themed baby clothes, *Psycho Baby*.

Today, Wicker Park is one of Chicago's thriving inner suburbs, named by *Forbes* magazine in 2014 as one of the US's top 10 'hippest neighbourhoods'. But its colonization by creatives means the Polish delis and Puerto Rican businesses once characteristic of the area have disappeared, with many of the previously impressive industrial buildings gutted and converted into the type of condos one can see in any gentrifying neighbourhood of Chicago (Makagon 2010). This confirms that 'promotion of the creative class, and its habitus, if not actively checked, is a de facto support for a particular type of gentrification, and an implicit, or often explicit, (re-) ordering of social and cultural priorities' (Pratt 2011: 296). This is also something that's been observed in perhaps the most infamous British example of arts-fuelled regeneration, Hoxton in East London. Artists started moving into this undesirable, socially disadvantaged area during the late 1980s and early 1990s when old warehouse spaces suitable for studios were available at cheap rent. These included some of the biggest names in contemporary British art: Damien Hirst, Gavin

Turk, Dinos and Jake Chapman, Rachel Whiteread, Chris Ofili, Gillian Wearing, Sarah Lucas and Tracey Emin (many of whom studied at Goldsmiths College, South London). Appropriating the working-class socio-cultural practices they observed in the area (Harris 2012), these young British artists challenged the perceived elitism of the London art scene via provocative exhibitions (notably the 1997 'Sensation' show). In turn, their activDities transformed the locale:

> Hoxton was invented in 1993. Before that, there was only 'Oxton, a scruffy no man's land of pie and mash and cheap market-stall clothing, a place where taxi drivers of the old school were proud to have been born but were reluctant to take you to. It did not register so much as a blip on the cultural radar. Hoxton, on the other hand, became the first great art installation of the Young British Artists: an urban playground tailor-made to annoy middle England, where everyone had scruffy clothes and daft haircuts and stayed up late, and no one had a proper job. By the end of the 90s, Hoxton had spawned an entire lifestyle: the skinhead had been replaced by the fashionable 'Hoxton fin' as the area's signature haircut, the derelict warehouses turned into million-pound lofts. As the groovy district *du jour*, Hoxton had come to represent the cliff-face of the cutting edge, and everyone wanted a piece. (Cartner-Morley 2003: 17)

Hoxton and the City fringes became home to a rich variety of trendy restaurants, boutiques, clubs and pubs in the 1990s and early 2000s. Long-established pubs such as the *Bricklayer's Arms* (Charlotte Street) and the *Betsey Trotwood* became renowned as spaces where artists mixed with media creatives, students and Britpop musicians, while new electro-clash clubs, galleries and fusion restaurants (*Cargo, 333, Swish, The Electricity Showrooms, Troy, 291 Gallery*, etc.) sprung up around Shoreditch and Hoxton. While this regeneration was, as Andy Pratt (2009) details, at best partial and selective, there's little question arts-led transformation turned much of this down-at-heel and marginalized district into a highly desirable residential and commercial location, ultimately pushing the artists out. By 2007, graffiti artist Banksy was drawing attention to the ongoing cleansing of the area, his 'Sweeping it Under the Carpet' mural on the side of jay Jopling's cutting-edge *White Cube* itself quickly disappearing under whitewash (Fig. 9.1).

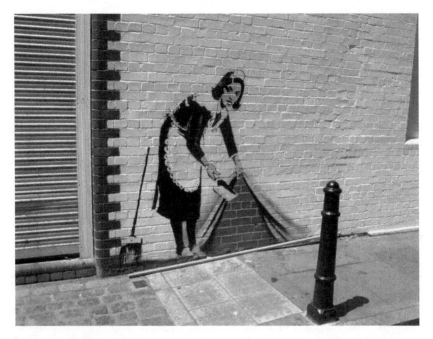

Fig. 9.1 Gentrifiying Hoxton: Banksy's (2007) stencil mural 'Sweeping it under the carpet' (photo: Matt Brown, Flickr, used under a CCBY license)

Andrew Harris (2012) concludes that Hoxton's story shows there's a 'field of gentrification' in which the cultural capital developed by artists through their 'valorisation of the mundane' is appropriated by market forces leading to the subsequent displacement of artists to cheaper districts. This is an interpretation that leans on David Ley's (2003) studies of arts-led gentrification in Vancouver, which suggested that inner city embourgeoisement was primarily manifest in the opening of antique shops, boutiques, French restaurants and galleries in districts that had been previously identified as lower status. For Ley, this indicated the pivotal role of artists in gentrification, with the perceived uplift of many neighbourhoods starting via the emergence of such artistic and 'bohemian' stores. However, Ley suggested these quickly began to be linked to other forms of 'creative capital', such as those associated with advertising, architecture and publishing. Within a few short years, this created a local service economy almost entirely oriented to upper middle-class populations, and one no longer affordable to artists.

The story of Hoxton and Young British Art is hence one that fits into this oft-told story of culture-led revivification and subsequent gentrification. The story goes something like this: in the first stage, a 'creative underclass' discovers a neighbourhood's special character, such as its social diversity, architectural heritage, specialist ethnic stores or vibrant street markets. Non-traditional 'footloose' individuals are particularly numerous, comprising members of urban subcultures, artists, students and 'dropouts'. These 'urban pioneers' make this run-down or even dangerous area more livable and attractive to other 'cool hunting' individuals who would not normally venture there—and, in so doing, encourage the beginnings of housing speculation (Smith 1996a, 1996b). Improvement by individuals is followed by entrepreneurial investment, and ultimately corporate speculation and middle-class gentrification. The edgy character of the area is lost as it drowns in a sea of overpriced craft beer and hand-roasted coffee: 'domestication by cappuccino', as Rowland Atkinson (2003: 1832) puts it.

In the wake of the 'regeneration maelstrom' following the 2012 London Olympics, inner London areas including Hoxton and Shoreditch—but also Brixton, Camden, Deptford and Peckham—have become highly contested spaces, with conflict essentially between two groups: 'the affluent gentrifiers and corporate businesses, and those (smaller firms, some residents, and visitors) who stand for the prominence of transgressive subcultures, and liminality' (Gornostaeva and Campbell 2012: 183). These conflicts are writ large in struggles over High Streets, which often appear on the frontline in struggles involving the transformation of the 'local' and authentic into a consumer spectacle. This is often ripe for satire. For example, in Paul Case's (2012) short story, 'The Battle of Kingsland Road', a gang of gentrifiers from Stoke Newington and the *fashionistas* of the Hoxton Liberation Army both claim Kingsland Road, Hackney, as their own, triggering a brutal turf war. But sometimes, the fact is as remarkable as the fiction. Shops once catering for less-affluent communities have been reinvented in accordance with the latest fads. Kingsland Road cannot quite match Bethnal Green Road's *Dinah's Cat Emporium*, where it's possible to drink tea surrounded by nine resident cats, but it does boast *Dream Bags, Jaguar Shoes* (a hipster bar that's taken over two neighbouring wholesale premises), alcoholic milkshake shacks,

Brazilian cocktail bars, vintage shops and Vietnamese *banh mi* sandwich shops. Round the corner, there's a burger and craft beer joint in the old Asian Women's Advisory Centre, the sign remaining above the door, and the menus ironically offering 'advice' on which burgers to pick (£7.50 for a buttermilk chicken burger with emmental and avocado). South of the river, in Deptford, hipster gentrification reached new heights of irony in 2014 with the opening of *The Job Centre*, a bar with a 'pop-up kitchen' that replaced a facility that local councilors had fought but failed to retain, despite rising local unemployment (Fig. 9.2).

These businesses, and others like them, attract a colourful range of commentary from those who feel the East End is not merely losing its character but being priced beyond the pockets of longer-established residents. For example, in 2014, the opening of the *Cereal Killers* café in Brick Lane, Tower Hamlets—a business selling imported cereals at

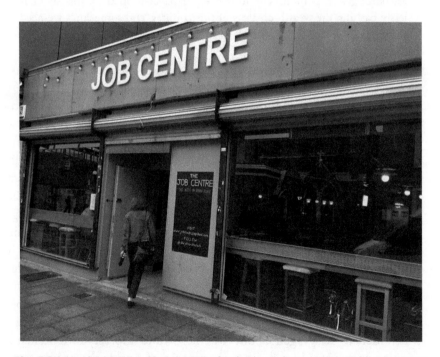

Fig. 9.2 Ironic consumption in Deptford: The Job Centre bar (photo: Matt Brown, Creative Commons CC BY)

premium prices—attracted critical headlines pointing out the disparity between this and the fact that 49 % of children in the local borough lived in poverty, many going without breakfast. This attack encouraged Boris Johnson, Mayor of London, to weigh in with his defence:

> *Channel Four* … sent a reporter to cover the story of the *Cereal Killers* café in Shoreditch—and he generally monstered the poor entrepreneurs. He was scathing about charging £2.50 minimum for a bowl of cereal; he mocked the proprietors—a gentle pair of bearded hipsters—for their pretensions to gentrify the area, and suggested that local people would not be able to eat there. He put the boot in, and I am not at all sure he was right to do so … We should be hailing anyone who starts a business in this country; we should acclaim them for overcoming all the obstacles that government puts in their path—the rates, the employment law, the health and safety. It's a great thing to want to open a place of work in one of the poorest boroughs in Britain. We don't need taxpayer-funded journalists endlessly bashing the wealth-creators of this country, and sometimes we need to be a little less cynical and a bit more encouraging. (Johnson 2014: np)

Yet, such appeals did not prevent the café being attacked in a 2015 Class War demonstration ('Fuck London'), which proclaimed on its *Facebook* page, 'We don't want luxury flats that no one can afford, we want genuinely affordable housing. We don't want pop-up gin bars or brioche buns—we want community'. Red paint and cereal were daubed on the windows, as the crowds shouted 'scum' at the owners and frightened clientele. In the wake of this, there was sustained discussion as to whether such hipster-run shabby chic businesses should bear the brunt of the anger of those who feel our cities are being taken away from working-class communities. For every person condemning the shop for driving the gentrification frontier further into working-class neighbourhoods, it seemed there were others leaping to its defence, proclaiming that independent businesses like *Cereal Killers* are actually the last bastion holding out against big businesses encroaching on the East End (see Gillan 2015).

Entrepreneurial urban pioneers or exploitative parasites? Or both? Much debate has raged about whether white hipster entrepreneurs opening businesses like this are a symptom of London's ensuing gentrification or causal agents. But gentrification is nothing but complex.

Certainly, hipster incomers are involved in the refiguring of local taste cultures, but they are not solely to blame for the processes making London neighbourhoods unaffordable for the less affluent. Crucially, there needs to be serious attention paid to the local authority policies encouraging the displacement of existing working-class communities, particularly stock transfer and the redevelopment of council estates by private developers (Lees 2014).

But a wealth of literature now confirms artists are deliberately used as avant-garde gentrifiers by real estate agents even if they do not act consciously as developers themselves. In Shoreditch, for instance, estate agents Stirling Ackroyd reputedly targeted adverts for short-life live/work leases at artists (who they termed 'scuzzers') in order to build a rental market and attract investment in property into the area. Ley (2003: 2541), hence excuses artists from any blame for gentrification, suggesting it's the 'societal valorization of the competencies of the artist that subsequently attracts followers richer in economic capital'. In this sense, it's possible to depict artists as victims of gentrification. Indeed, once artists are established in former cultural 'wastelands' they create little oases of hipster-attracting cool, slowly pushing away the ethnic and class diversity that made the area affordable in the first place. And herein lies the problem. As Deb Cowen (2006: 22) writes, once upon a time hipsters might have been considered as those 'who were readily displaced the moment people with financial capital' stepped in, but today they 'are actively working to institutionalize themselves in the city'. Suggesting that 'they have recently found allies in government and business who see possibilities of accumulation by good design', Cowen continues to suggest they have become agents of neoliberalism, colonizing the inner city and claiming it as their own through 'banal, mimetic, creativity'. Hipsterfication is no longer the prelude to gentrification, it is gentrification.

At this stage, it's worth repeating that retail gentrification is centrally implicated in these processes of 'creative destruction' in the sense it revalues vacant properties and at the same time it sends out signals to potential residents and investors that particular neighbourhoods are ripe for reinvention. The emergence of cool or 'crunchy' consumer spaces where the distinction can be displayed makes these neighbourhoods more attractive not just to creative workers looking for a livable working environment, but to other potential incomers who want their lives to feel unique and edgy (Makagon 2010). Creative city policies and retail change are thus closely related, both potentially turning 'authentic inner city liminality' into gentrified spectacle. While some working-class tastes and cultures can be appropriated to these ends, the cultural valorization of particular aesthetic and cultural forms over others encourages displacement and dispossession: gradual changes in the aesthetic and performative codes of the neighbourhood begin to affect some peoples' ability to participate in everyday life and slowly the area becomes inaccessible to long-term dwellers. The fact these changes are typically non-catastrophic and incremental indicates what Leslie Kern (2015b) terms the 'slow violence' of gentrification. Perhaps it's this that explains the lack of overt resistance to such processes, albeit activists like Paul Case have sought to draw attention to them through forms of DIY urbanism:

> I lived in and helped run a squatted social centre called *Well Furnished* on Well Street [*South Hackney*] in 2011, where we had strong links with the local residents and traders who were fighting against ludicrous rent inflations. The same property managers and owners who were inflating these rents were the ones who managed and owned the connected shops we had occupied. Naturally, we became a small part of the history of that struggle, as it was an embarrassment to the owners that buildings they'd left to rot were being put to positive use. We ran poetry and music events, ran workshops and let other groups use the space for their activities and meetings, and all for free or on a donation basis. I don't think this was the redevelopment that the owners had in mind, but it was definitely better than having a *Starbucks* there. (Case 2013: np)

Elsewhere, squatters similarly occupied a café on Broadway Market in 2005, fighting the demolition of the *Francesca Café*, a much-used local facility that was open for 30 years, but slated for redevelopment as 'yuppie flats'. This politicized occupation of a vacant retail space contrasts nicely with the anodyne use of retail units for pop-up shops selling Christmas cards or community crafts goods (Harris 2015). But it's all too rare, and, arguably, it's taken the plight of the E15 mothers—a group of social housing residents being forcibly rehoused by Newham Council—to really draw attention to the spatial injustices of gentrification in the East

End of London. It's telling that the Carpenters' Estate, from which they are threatened with removal, is only a stone's throw from the Stratford Westfield Shopping Centre, as well as the emerging 'cultural district' on the former Olympic park, intended to host two museums, the Sadlers' Wells dance theatre and the University of Arts London campus.

Bohemia By the Sea?

While evidence from London and elsewhere shows that arts-based regeneration can trigger gentrification in retail and residential environments alike, the idea that art is good for the High Street is hard to shake off. Pop-up galleries and community art spaces have become a widespread visual and performative 'filler' of urban vacancy, especially in Portas pilot towns (Ferreri 2016). One reason for this is that the artist is imagined as an agent of positive renewal, an 'independent' actor who is not solely motivated by profit. The anti-bourgeois and anti-conformist disposition of the artist makes it hard to reconcile art-led regeneration with gentrification, as artists are often publically disdainful about the commodification of art. Instead, they frequently proclaim to find value in the commonplace, and revel in the grittier and seamier sides of urban life (Harris 2012). Unlike corporate-led gentrification, the colonization of space by artists is not necessarily seen as the precursor to the introduction of mimetic serialized middle-class culture, but the inverse of that (Makagon 2010). This given, the emergence of 'bohemian' businesses or galleries on the High Street is broadly welcomed because they are discoursed as 'local', counter-posed with the global brandscapes found on many High Streets.

Originally referring to the spaces of nineteenth-century art production in Paris, the label bohemia carries with it a romanticized imaginary of freewheeling, countercultural experimentation and excess (see Wilson 2000). This is often contrasted with the lifestyle and spaces of the bourgeoisie, who favour a more Protestant work ethic and adhere to a more respectable set of moral codes and conventions. The distinct 'structures of feeling' created in bohemian retail spaces thus proclaim the main elements of what Henri Lefebvre (1991) termed 'differential' space: space created and dominated by its users through bodily practices which value quality over quantity, the look over the gaze and the sensual over the scientific. Bohemian businesses also appear to be 'free zones' whose functional and economic role is sometimes difficult to explain in terms of capitalist economics (Groth and Corijn 2005). Indeed, the proprietors of many independent galleries, micropubs and real coffee shops appear outwardly indifferent to notions of profit, sometimes being portrayed as enthusiastic 'curators' rather than astute business people (Hracs et al. 2013). Aesthetically and practically, bohemian businesses hence exude a lazy, emancipatory 'urbanity'—albeit a form of urbanism highly valued by those consumers who place a premium on scarcity and the 'one-off'. The relationship between the bourgeois and bohemian is consequently full of ambiguity, with the former often extending their influence into the spaces of the latter as they use their financial capital to purchase cultural capital.

One implication is that bohemian spaces are short-lived, as they are quickly incorporated into a more conventional set of practices as the bourgeoisie move in. Or perhaps the distinction between these—like that between the artist and the hipster—is no longer relevant in the city of the twenty-first century? Whatever, the outcome is often the creation of a pseudo-bohemia, a bobo (i.e. bohemian-bourgeois) space. As the example of Hoxton suggests, the media popularization of 'edgy' artistic quarters can lead to increased commercial interest in such areas and generate spiralling property prices that displace the 'original' creative pioneers (very often low-income street artists, ethnic minorities or queer-identified populations). As Rebecca Solnit (2000) laments, part of what makes a city really vital and stimulating, and what really gets the creative juices flowing, is the braiding together of disparate lives and diverse cultures, something threatened by a gentrification which severs some of these strands completely, diminishing urbanism itself. As she argues, Bohemia has been all but driven out of Manhattan as the last pockets of poverty got gentrified in the closing decades of the twentieth century, and hipster districts like Wicker Park, Pioneer Square (Seattle) and Williamsburg (Brooklyn) threaten to go the same way. But what, if anything, does this imply for those towns on the English margins seeking to revive their fortunes—and their High Streets—through arts-based regeneration?

As we have seen, Margate became a Portas Pilot town in 2012. But several years before Mary Portas, Queen of Shops, arrived to sprinkle her magic retail dust on the High Street, Margate was already being vaunted as undergoing a culture-fuelled revival, with the Arts Council of England proclaiming 'Margate is a great example of how art can play an effective role in regeneration' (ACE 2009), with the Margate Renewal Strategy (2008) having been explicit about aiming to turn the town into a hub for cultural events, artistic goods and 'creative production'. Much of the impetus here was provided by plans for the Turner Contemporary gallery, mooted as early as 1994 as a means of capitalizing on the fact that JWM Turner (1775–1881) had lived in Margate as a child and returned in later life, completing at least a hundred paintings around the Kent coast. Although planning permission for the gallery, designed by Snohetta and Spence, was granted in 2003, with the intention of this being a spectacular fin-like construction on the harbour arm, initial survey and scoping work suggested that the costs could rise to as much as £50 million—well above the original estimate of £7 million. Following litigation, a change of plans saw the architect David Chipperfield designing a simpler, shed-like structure, very similar to his design for Wakefield's Hepworth Gallery but intended to capture the daylight of the north-facing Kent coast. This gallery opened in 2011, at a cost of £17.5 million to Kent County Council and partners. By 2013, it had welcomed a million visitors, attracted by initial exhibits including one from Margate-born 'Young British Artist' Tracey Emin and another by walking artist Hamish Fulton (there's no permanent collection at the Turner).

But the lack of a permanent venue before 2011 did not prevent the Turner Contemporary actively commissioning art. Much of this addressed issues directly relevant to the regeneration of Margate—and 'quality of life issues' (Pomery 2013: 16)—at a time when the national press was beginning to pick up on the movement of significant numbers of Roma and Eastern European migrants into some of the areas known for defunct B&Bs and subdivided holiday lets (sample headline in *The Daily Express*, 2004: 'Flood of Immigrants makes township ghettos of Britain's seaside'). The Arrivals project in 2005, for instance, involved artists from the eight Eastern European nations that had just joined the EU, while in 2006, the Unite project bought young French artists to Margate at the same time that two British artists, Bob and Roberta Smith, oversaw the *Should I Stay or Should I Go?* initiative which saw the hanging of colourful banners along Margate High Street posing rhetorical questions: 'Britain or Brittany? The Arctic Monkeys or Mantovani? Kent or Cornwall?' Other projects also explored Margate's attempts to deal with issues of immigration, with London-based arts group Artangel commissioning a number of artists to collaborate in a one-day arts-based festival, *Exodus* (2006). Part of this was the hanging of banner portraits around the town of 22 children who had come to Margate from Congo, Iraqi, Egypt and Eastern Europe. This *Towards a Promised Land* project also saw Wendy Eward working with these young people to produce their own art, ultimately hung in a local gallery (Balfour 2014). The centerpiece, however, was an immersive piece of street theatre centred around the re-telling of the Book of Exodus in which the tale of one man's attempts to banish refugees, drug users and the homeless from his kingdom culminated in the burning of sculptor Anthony Gormley's 25-metre high *Waste Man* in the grounds of the (then) defunct *Dreamland* fun fair. This sculpture was constructed from the detritus of modern consumer society—planks of wood, tables, paintings, chairs, keyboards, dartboards, a front door, toilet seats—all donated by local people. In much of the media, this event was seen as an exuberant launch party for the coming cultural regeneration of the town, with plans for the rebuilding of *Dreamland* as a 'retro' amusement park further suggesting room for optimism.

The 2008 document, *A Cultural Vision for Margate: The Next Ten Years*, commissioned by the Margate Renewal partnership, underscored this commitment to produce a 'creative Margate' (Ward 2016). This document spoke of embedding the Turner Contemporary in a creative community that would contribute to a distinctive Margate 'brand' by combining seaside heritage with a 'cultural narrative', but also insisted Margate must be a town where 'culture is for everyone'. Putting art on the High Street was a key part of this, with the acquisition of the former *Marks and Spencer* store by Thanet District Council (at a cost of some £4.5 million) providing the Turner Contemporary a temporary home. Other vacant shops were also enlivened, with the 2009 *Window of Opportunity* project overseen by Emily Firmin (daughter of famed children's animator Peter

Firmin) filling empty shop fronts with papier-mâché art suggesting how these premises might be used in the future. Counting down to the opening of the Turner Contemporary proper, the Council put further money into tackling 'eyesore' buildings between the train station and the gallery by working with the owners of empty shops to develop innovative solutions to bring them back into use, particularly working with artists. Heather Sawney, arts development officer for Thanet District Council, led this, initially as part of the 'Margate Rocks' art festival. In her view, what changed was that instead of petitioning reluctant property owners for short, low-cost rentals, artists became embraced. As she explained, 'what art can do is show that there really is still a use for these spaces and that's useful to property owners and to the community'.

There's no question this embedding of art in the townscape, and the buzz associated with the cultural activities led by the Turner Contemporary (as well as smaller arts organizations including Limbo and Crate), has had a transformational effect on the town's reputation. But it's the palpable changes to the streets near the Turner, in the Old Town, that have attracted most attention, its mix of cafés, vintage shops and boutiques being presented as evidence of cultural renaissance:

> Margate [once] felt like a brutish, irredeemable place but last summer I'd heard enough positive mentions of it to make me wonder whether this seaside town that had been in freefall for as long as anyone could remember had finally found its bounce: conversations turned on its new "arty" vibe, people moving there, people even calling it "Shoreditch-on-Sea" … Men in sharp black Harrington jackets with tartan lining, sideburned and mod-cropped, were drinking pints that glowed amber in the sun outside a bar proudly displaying a Northern Soul fist and a Trojan Records logo on its front … They looked fucking cool, too: an alternative style cult … up-cycling that old spirit of south coast youth culture that Margate was a midwife to. This side street into the Old Town showed a … decidedly more bourgeois side to this retro-modernist current bubbling away in Margate: a mid-century Danish furniture shop, a craft beer pub, a "Delivery to London" sign in a yard with vintage bath tubs and Seventies reclining chairs. Gift shops and do-up-your-new-house-stylishly stores, as sure a sign as the Farrow & Ball-coloured estate agents that this end of Margate was coming "up". (Smith 2015: np)

The idea Margate is a 'sandy hipster paradise' has clearly caught on, with the Rough Guide 2012 proclaiming Margate one of the world's top 10 must-see locations. Travel writers have extolled the town's combination of dilapidated seaside charm and artful venues in Sunday supplements and style sheets galore. Some of these hyperbolic accounts have been greeted with a degree of local incredulity, but in 2013 the independent think tank, the Centre for Social Justice (2013: 17), concluded the Turner Contemporary had 'helped signal a change in attitudes'. Walking from the station to the Turner Contemporary on a blisteringly hot Saturday in July 2015 to visit Grayson Perry's *Provincial Punk* exhibit, I begin to believe this. Margate is packed, the sands busy with sunbathers, the whole beach swaying to the sounds of a Caribbean sound system down from London. Dreamland's been open for just three weeks, and it's the first time I have seen its bold neon signs imploring visitors to visit. Admittedly, as I walk along the front, there are still empty businesses but I note that one facing the clock tower that has been boarded up for years has been adorned with new street art, one a funky mural bizarrely featuring goth musician Nick Cave, another in the pop art style of Roy Lichtenstein, another of a mermaid. All the seats outside the bars in the Old Town are taken, sunburnt and tattooed bodies on display. The Grayson Perry show is busy, groups shuffling round the cool interior of the Turner in due reverence, and there are even large numbers on the High Street itself, some attracted perhaps by the band proclaiming the opening of the newest boutique (*Affordable Art*) in *Pop-up Margate*, initially opened by Mary Portas in 2012 as *Poportunity* (Fig. 9.3). I end the day drinking cocktails served in jam jars in a small bar above the Tom Thumb theatre, following a gig and film screening organized by the owner of local *Forts Café* (a retro hipster diner selling burgers and sandwiches made from local Kentish ingredients).

All this seems like *prima facie* evidence of the 'Turner Effect', and the ability of culture-led regeneration to kick-start something significant. The town seemed much more vibrant place compared with the, admittedly rather grey, day in 2012 when I'd been in town for Mary Portas' launching of the Town Team initiative. In the interim, I'd often have conversations with lecturer friends from Canterbury and Whitstable who would drop into conversations how they'd found this great new pizza place in

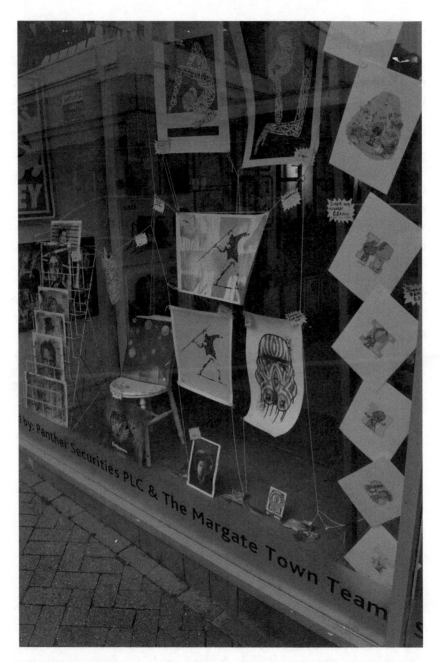

Fig. 9.3 Affordable art and Banksy reproductions in the window of the 'Pop-up Margate' shop (photo: author)

Margate—of all places!—or tell me about a great reclamation yard where the owner would deliver pieces of 1950s furniture to anywhere in Kent for free. Clearly, the changing retail offer of the Old Town has proved a significant draw, giving visitors and the 'Down from Londons' something to do once they spent their obligatory 30 minutes or so in the Turner. The publicity surrounding the Wayne Hemingway-designed *Dreamland* has been another important fillip for the town, with this retro amusement park making up for a lack of white-knuckle rides with refitted vintage attractions, restyled for modern audiences (including a 'Counter-Culture Caterpillar' ride and spinning Wedgwood tea cups). This new-found confidence has been mirrored in a 2015 £330,000 award from the Arts Council to the Turner Contemporary and Kent County Council (alongside other partners) as part of the Cultural Destinations programme, intended to increase visitor numbers to the county by 5% over three years.

So Margate seems to be beginning to carve out a new identity, no longer known solely as a faded seaside town but one that combines retro chic, cheeky seaside fun, designer cool and edgy bohemianism. The fact it's 'rough round the edges', and far from polished, is part of its appeal. But, crucially, it's not been for everyone. Some local artists are highly ambivalent about the changes they have witnessed:

> The current "contemporary" management at Turner has from the moment it started alienated locals by a steadfast refusal to support local artists—they would say otherwise! I was told when asking for a week a year for local artists that "I do not want Sunday afternoon artists in an international gallery". I have myself been to the gallery and have been bitterly disappointed. There have obviously been some creative admissions figures published but for my own part the views fed back show that it's not helping regenerate the town but I would be pleased if proved wrong. I have seen this nation-wide and it's a complete waste of public money, which we no longer have. (Michael Wheatley-Ward, Fellow of the Royal Society for Arts, cited in Lees and McKiernan 2012: 30)

Likewise, Jon Ward (2015: 214) cites Pat, an artist with a studio in Margate, who contends 'the overriding concern of the local and county councils with regards to the Turner Contemporary is that while it's making money and they're getting the kudos from it, I don't see local artists still getting much of a look in'. However, others are more ambivalent and understand why the gallery is using 'big name' artists to attract visitors to the town. Those with small galleries in the town are at least happy to pick up some passing trade. But there's certainly an implicit danger that the showcasing of 'international' rather than local artists at the Turner consolidates an imagined divide between 'creative' incomers and existing residents, especially those from Margate's less advantaged ethnic minority populations, whom, the Director of the Turner, Victoria Pomeroy has publically acknowledged, have not shown much interest in visiting the gallery. Indeed, despite her well-intentioned belief in the redemptive and transformative qualities of art, I have cringed listening to her talking about the need to 'educate' Margate residents into appreciating the art at the Turner Contemporary. Ward (2015) also cites artists and visitors who refer to a gentrified bubble of creative activity in the town, and a 'wilderness' beyond. This type of talk ultimately divides the so-called *creative class*, deemed to have the capacity to engage with designated creative spaces and the 'uncreative' classes who populate the more 'ordinary' city (Edensor et al. 2009).

So even if Margate High Street is beginning to benefit from arts-based regeneration, it's mainly through a slow creep of gentrified businesses out of the Old Town into the vacant shops now ripe for incoming entrepreneurs, like the owners of the boutique *Sands* hotel or the small-scale producers who hawk graffiti art, craft soaps and retro computer games in the pop-up shop. But although it now boasts such obviously gentrified consumer spaces, central Margate and adjacent wards remain relatively deprived, the periphery of London's ridiculously overheated core. It's not clear whether those living in the overcrowded flats and bedsits of north Margate and Cliftonville have any particular use for overpriced craft goods or 'affordable art'. The solution to the many vacancies on Margate's High Street—making the street more attractive to the creative and cognitive class by providing pop-up shops, boutiques and leisured retailing—is then slowly 'bringing it back to life'. But it's important to remember it was never dead, even if it's haunted by the memories of what it used to be. Margate High Street was, at the height of the recession, a poor High Street catering predominantly to poor people.

There's then a very real possibility that many of those have long used Margate High Street for both sociality and shopping will find themselves increasingly marginalized on a High Street that is being reinvented in line with the visions typified by the nostalgic boho-chic worldview offered by Mary Portas. The emergent High Street might be in keeping with the tastes and dispositions of those down from London and elsewhere in the Home Counties to visit the Turner Contemporary, but whether it fulfills the needs of all local residents is moot: retail gentrification will surely be accompanied by residential gentrification, the dispossessed moved on again. While this type of hypothesis currently lacks empirical substantiation—the High Street remains a work in progress—it's already possible to question whether the outcome will be the creation of a vibrant, mixed-used street that caters to the many, or a more select one that prospers on the back of more affluent and discerning consumption. Ultimately, the arts-based regeneration of Margate High Street may be judged a success, but whether this is at the cost of displacement, exclusion and gentrification remains to be seen.

References

Arts Council England. (2009). Making over Margate. Retrieved from http://www.artscouncil.org.uk/news/arts-council-news/making-over-margate/

Atkinson, R. (2003). Domestication by cappuccino or a revenge on urban space? Control and empowerment in the management of public spaces. *Urban Studies, 40*(9), 1829–1843.

Balfour, M. (2014). Performing the promised land: The festivalizing of multicultures in the Margate Exodus Project. In I. Woodward, J. Taylor, & A. Bennett (Eds.), *The festivalization of culture*. Farnham: Ashgate.

Bridge, G. (2006). It's not just a question of taste: Gentrification, the neighbourhood, and cultural capital. *Environment and Planning A, 38*(10), 1965–1985.

Cameron, S., & Coaffee, J. (2005). Art, gentrification and regeneration—From artist as pioneer to public arts. *European Journal of Housing Policy, 5*(1), 39–58.

Cartner-Morley, J. (2003). Where have all the cool people gone? *The Guardian*, 21 November, http://www.theguardian.com/lifeandstyle/2003/nov/21/fashion1

Case, P. (2013). Interview with Paul Case. http://www.influxpress.com/author-interviews/paul_case/

Case, P. (2012). The battle of Kingsland Road. In G. Budden & K. Caless (Eds.), *Acquired for development: A Hackney anthology*. London: Influx Press.

Centre for Social Justice (2013). *Turning the tide: Social justice in five seaside towns*. London: Centre for Social Justice.

Chang, T. C. (2016). New uses need old buildings: Gentrification aesthetics and the arts in Singapore. *Urban Studies, 53*(3), 524–539.

Cowen, D. (2006). Hipster urbanism. *Relay*, September/October, 22–25.

Department for Culture, Media and Sports (DCMS) (2001). *Creative industries mapping document*. London: DCMS.

Edensor, T., Leslie, D., Millington, S., & Rantisi, N. (Eds.) (2009). *Spaces of vernacular creativity: Rethinking the cultural economy*. Routledge: London.

Ferreri, M. (2016). Pop-up shops as interruptions in (post-) recessional London. In J. Shirley and C. Lindner (eds) *Cities interrupted. Visual Culture and Urban Space*. London, Bloomsbury.

Florida, R. (2002). *The rise of the creative class*. New York: Basic Books.

Gillan, A. (2015). The Hipster Cereal Killer Café owners aren't the East End's real enemy. *The Guardian*, 27 September, http://www.theguardian.com/commentisfree/2015/sep/27/hipster-cereal-killer-cafe-gentrification-east-end

Gornostaeva, G., & Campbell, N. (2012). The creative underclass in the production of place: Example of Camden Town in London. *Journal of Urban Affairs, 34*(2), 169–188.

Groth, J., & Corijn, E. (2005). Reclaiming urbanity: Indeterminate spaces, informal actors and urban agenda setting. *Urban Studies, 42*(3), 503–526.

Harris, A. (2012). Art and gentrification: Pursuing the urban pastoral in Hoxton, London. *Transactions of the Institute of British Geographers, 37*(2), 226–241.

Harris, E. (2015). Navigating pop-up geographies: Urban space–times of flexibility, interstitiality and immersion. *Geography Compass, 9*(11), 592–603.

Harvie, J. (2013). *Fair play: Art, performance and neoliberalism*. Palgrave Macmillan: Basingstoke.

Haylett, C. (2001). Illegitimate subjects? Abject whites, neoliberal modernisation and middle class multiculturalism. *Environment and Planning D: Society and Space., 19*(3), 351–370.

Hracs, B. J., Jakob, D., & Hauge, A. (2013). Standing out in the crowd: The rise of exclusivity-based strategies to compete in the contemporary marketplace for music and fashion. *Environment and Planning A, 45*(5), 1144–1161.

Jayne, M. (2005). *Cities and consumption*. London: Routledge.

Johnson, B. (2014). Don't murder the cereal killers—We need people just like them. *The Daily Telegraph*, 15 December. http://www.telegraph.co.uk/comment/11293491/Dont-murder-the-Cereal-Killers-we-need-people-just-like-them.html

Kern, L. (2015b). Rhythms of gentrification: Eventfulness and slow violence in a happening neighbourhood. Cultural Geographies, 1474474015591489.

Landry, C., & Bianchini, F. (1995). *The creative city*. London: Demos.

Latham, A. (2003). Urbanity, lifestyle and making sense of the new urban cultural economy: Notes from Auckland, New Zealand. *Urban Studies, 40*(9), 1699–1724.

Lees, L. (2014). The urban injustices of new Labour's "New Urban Renewal": The case of the Aylesbury Estate in London. *Antipode, 46*(4), 921–947.

Lees, L., & McKiernan, J. (2012). Art-led regeneration in Margate: Learning from Moonbow Jakes Café and Lido nightclub intervention. *Art & the Public Sphere, 2*(1-3), 17–35.

Lefebvre, H. (1991). *The production of space*. Oxford: Blackwell.

Ley, D. (2003). Artists, aestheticisation and the field of gentrification. *Urban Studies, 40*(12), 2527–2544.

Lloyd, R. (2002). Neo–bohemia: Art and neighborhood redevelopment in Chicago. *Journal of Urban Affairs, 24*(5), 517–532.

Makagon, D. (2010). Bring on the shock troops: Artists and gentrification in the popular press. *Communication and Critical/Cultural Studies, 7*(1), 26–52.

Margate Renewal Strategy. (2008). *A cultural vision for Margate: Creative Margate ten year delivery plan*. Margate: Margate Renewal Partnership.

Mathews, V. (2014). Incoherence and tension in culture-led redevelopment. *International Journal of Urban and Regional Research, 38*(3), 1019–1036.

O'Connor, J. (2000). The definition of the 'cultural industries'. *The European Journal of Arts Education, 2*(3), 15–27.

Peck, J. (2005). Struggling with the creative class. *International journal of urban and regional research, 29*(4), 740–770.

Peck, J. (2012). Austerity urbanism: American cities under extreme economy. *City, 16*(6), 626–655.

Perry, G. (2013). Reith lectures 2013: Playing to the gallery. Transcript of Radio 4 transmission, 29 October. http://downloads.bbc.co.uk/radio4/transcripts/reith-lecture3-londonderry.pdf

Pomery, V. (2013). Selling culture to Margate. *Context, 80*, 15–16.

Pratt, A. C. (2009). Urban regeneration: From the arts 'feel good' factor to the cultural economy: A case study of Hoxton, London. *Urban Studies, 46*(5-6), 1041–1061.

Pratt, A. C. (2011). The cultural contradictions of the creative city. *City, Culture and Society, 2*(3), 123–130.

Rankin, K. N., & McLean, H. (2015). Governing the commercial streets of the city: New terrains of disinvestment and gentrification in Toronto's inner suburbs. *Antipode, 47*(1), 216–233.

Schlack, E., & Turnbull, N. (2015). Emerging retail gentrification in Santiago de Chile: The case of Italia-Caupolicán. In L. Lees, H. B. Shin, & E. Lopez-Morales (Eds.), *Global gentrifications: Uneven development and displacement.* Bristol: Policy Press.

Smith, M. (2015). How Margate became the new hipster's paradise. Esquire, 3 April, http://www.esquire.co.uk/food-drink/travel/8101/how-margate-became-the-new-hipsters-paradise/

Smith, N. (1996). *New urban frontier: Gentrification and the Revanchist City.* London: Routledge.

Solnit, R. (2000). *Hollow city.* New York: Verso.

Ward, J. (2015). *Cultural labour in the context of urban regeneration: Artists' work in Margate and Folkestone.* Doctoral thesis: University of Kent.

Ward, J. (2016). Down by the sea: Visual arts, artists and coastal regeneration. *International Journal of Cultural Policy.* doi:10.1080/10286632.2016.1153080.

Wilson, E. (2000). *Bohemians: The glamorous outcasts.* London: IB Tauris.

Zukin, S. (1995). *The cultures of cities.* Oxford: Blackwells.

10

Conclusion: Vital and Viable?

In this book, Mary Portas' review of High Streets, commissioned by the British government in 2011, has been taken to encapsulate much that appears to be taken as axiomatic in current thinking about the High Street. In this review, she argued the British High Street was declining alarmingly. For her, this was about more than simply the shift of retailing out of town and online, concerning the decline of community, and the evisceration of urban life:

> I believe that our High Streets have reached a crisis point. I believe that unless urgent action is taken much of Britain will lose, irretrievably, something that is fundamental to our society. Something that has real social as well as economic worth to our communities and that after many years of erosion, neglect and mismanagement, something I felt was destined to disappear forever. (Portas 2011: 2)

The revival of the High Street, as Portas stressed, appears fundamental in the creation of a sense of identity, 'giving back to the community a vibrant sense of belonging and place that will instill public respect and trust and a resource in times of personal or neighbourhood need' (Portas 2011: 3). The idea here is that if people no longer meet, trade and shop

© The Editor(s) (if applicable) and The Author(s) 2017
P. Hubbard, *The Battle for the High Street*,
DOI 10.1057/978-1-137-52153-8_10

on High Streets around the country, something important—perhaps indefinable—will be lost. As Portas (2011: 3) continues 'I believe that our High Streets are a really important part of building communities and pulling people together in a way that a supermarket or shopping mall, however convenient, however entertaining and however slick, just never can'.

While Portas' report was dismissed in some quarters as backward-looking (see especially Grimsey 2013), her views have been echoed in innumerable government policy statements. For example, in its summary of the measures taken to revive the High Street, the Department of Communities and Local Government stated:

> Today, traditional High Streets are under threat not just from the growth of Internet shopping, but also out-of-town shopping. There are also concerns about the so-called 'clone town' phenomenon, with local character being lost as major chains dominate the High Street. This matters. If High Streets are left to wither, that leaves a hollow space running right through the heart of our communities; where there should be a bustling, thriving place for people to gather. (DCLG 2013: 3)

Such statements emphasizing the 'hollowing out' of the British High Street can easily be supported with reference to 'objective' indicators illustrating its decline. For example, statistics show the number of vacant retail properties has increased dramatically since the onset of the most recent recession in 2009 (at around 10,000 per year nationally) and that the overall number of sales on the High Street have decreased markedly (by around 4% between 2011 and 2014). At the same time, the rise of 'toxic' stores has been documented, with much emphasis given to the proliferation of bookmakers, discount stores, sex shops, takeaways and other 'unhealthy' outlets seen to encourage consumption of dubious worth.

The 'official' policy line on High Streets in Britain is then that they are not what they used to be, and risk obsolescence if something is not done to reverse their fortunes. But, as we have seen, the High Street is something of an empty signifier, being populated with significant meaning according to one's own experience and memories of particular times and spaces. The High Street cannot be considered a discrete place, and needs to be understood as an example of what Rob Shields (1991: 31) terms a socio-spatialization—a term he uses to designate 'the ongoing construction of the spatial at the level of the imaginary'. As he shows, collective imaginaries and mythologies combine with interventions in the landscape itself to name objects of study, and concretize them in thought, language and praxis. A socio-spatialization can then be considered as virtual, albeit it exhibits a virtuality that is manifest materially, discursively and in policy terms as the frame through which particular spatial problems—such as the decline of the 'Great British' High Street—can be understood.

Here, Shields' term resonates with Henri Lefebvre's ideas concerning the social production of space, which have become widely popularized in the social sciences as part of the putative 'spatial turn'. Henri Lefebvre's (1991) theorization of the production of space identified it as involving the interaction between perceived, conceived, and lived space, where perceived space refers to the relatively objective, concrete space of spatial practice; conceived space refers to mental constructions of space, creative ideas and representations of space and lived space is the physical deciphering and experience of both perceived and conceived space, also known as representational space. For Lefebvre, producing space necessarily involves reproducing the social relations bound up in it. As he insists, the production of urban space entails much more than just planning the material space of the city; it involves the production, reproduction and regulation of all aspects of its social life.

The beauty of Lefebvre's formulation is that it allows us to see the production of space as neither imposed 'from above' or created 'from below': it opens the social imagination to the ways space is made simultaneously in different registers, all of which need to be examined if we are to understand the socially contested nature of space, and its continual becoming. It also allows us to avoid the dangers of producing accounts of the city which repress the agency of those who live and experience the city at 'street level': the implicit danger in focusing on 'official' or sanctioned discourses of the High Street—such as those enshrined in policy documents—is that we perpetuate a partial account of urban life, a story told by intellectuals and for intellectuals which ignores the complex ways 'ordinary' citizens engage with, and change the city in the realms of everyday life (see Hubbard 2006). In relation to the High Street, this implies we need to examine not just the debates surrounding it but also in the memories, stories and actions of those urban dwellers that construct the story of the High Street at street level. This type of insight, with all it implies about the value of ethnographic research on shops, shoppers and shopping (see Hall 2012), also discourages what might be seen as a purely capital-centric approach, where the rhythms of the High Street are seen to be increasingly dictated by global processes, and dominated by retail capital.

It's in this sense that this book has approached local shopping streets as relational spaces, always contested and constituted through multiple spatial registers, including everyday practice. In doing so, it has refuted the assumption that High Streets are in terminal demise, suggesting this needs reconsideration in the light of the varied social and cultural roles these continue to play, particularly in the lives of the residualized working-class inhabitants whose voices are often silenced in media and policy debates. Here, it has echoed Suzanne Hall (2011: 2572), who argues that consideration of the social and cultural role of the High Street is particularly important in a context where 'economic measures of value will prevail over social ones, and more predictable store formats and brands may well be regarded as more viable than independent or ethnic shops'. Indeed, despite some recent attempts to consider the mundane and everyday consumption of local shopping streets, and the way this is inflected by class and identity (e.g. Hall 2011; Findlay and Sparks 2012; Townshend 2016), it appears the majority of research on British High Streets remains focused on the economic viability of its retail function alone (e.g. Wrigley and Dolega 2011) or else critically considers the security measures taken to attract back the affluent (e.g. Coleman 2004; Atkinson 2003). In contrast, few have taken the time to consider who has the 'right' to the High Street, evaluating different claims about the vitality and viability of High Streets with reference to the different social constituencies and populations who lay claim to this space.

It's for this reason this book set out to question the assumptions underpinning the regeneration of the British High Street. It's not been against regeneration per se. Clearly, the closure of stores and the spate of vacancies on many High Streets has been devastating for many local economies, and it's hard to argue against the need to bring such properties back into viable use. Pop-up shops, boutiques and gallery spaces, rented at low cost and sometimes on short-term leases, certainly enliven the retail landscape and provide visual interest in streets where lively frontages can help to encourage footfall. Micropubs, gourmet burger bars, real coffee shops and pop-up art galleries are certainly all preferable to empty shops, and, like Farmers' Markets, can counter the centrifugal attraction of out of town retail by offering a more bespoke, individual and 'authentic' shopping experience. As such, this book has not represented a critique of the principle of High Street regeneration per se. But it has questioned whether the generally proposed measures intended to secure regeneration are appropriately matched to the needs of those currently most reliant on the High Street, those least able, or reluctant, to use Internet shopping or drive out of town.

The main conclusion of this book is that 'official' visions of resilient, sustainable and vibrant High Streets are shaped by particular classed assumptions. In this respect, it seems there's a wholesale rejection of the idea that more betting shops, lap dance clubs, fast food outlets, discount shops or moneylenders might provide any sort of basis for making a High Street which has vitality and viability. All can create jobs, and constitute viable businesses. But all are evidently seen as deleterious, and even dirty, associated with ideas of 'immoral' or 'bad' consumption. Seemingly, policy-makers would rather have empty properties than these. As we have seen, policy-makers endlessly debate how to use planning and licensing laws to clamp down on the 'proliferation' of these noxious and undesirable businesses. This, I have argued, actually has little to do with risky or unhealthy behaviour, and everything to do with class-based prejudice against the poor in a society 'where outright contempt is freely expressed against the working class' (Skeggs 2009: 637). Indeed, High Street policy appears based on the belief that retail revival requires the return of the more affluent, not the matching of premises to the needs of existing users. Evidentially, there's no place for cheap goods on the High Street, as cheapness has become equated with dirt and disgust.

Considering the current range of attempts to renew and re-invent the British High Street, this Chapter concludes this book by challenging some of the more conventional attempts to measure the performance of town centres such as vacancy rates and commercial yields (e.g. Ravenscroft 2000). Arguing for a widened conception of the High Street as a sustainable space of economic and social reproduction—and noting that around two-thirds of trips to High Streets are for forms of exchange and interaction other than shopping (High Street London 2010)—this Chapter argues there's a strong case for resisting retail gentrification, arguing instead for the maintenance of streets that serve the poorest in society, as well as the more affluent. But this last Chapter begins by posing a more fundamental question: why is so little said about retail gentrification in Britain?

The Gentrification of the Mind?

Writing in 2006, Tom Slater argued the literature on urban gentrification was becoming increasingly redundant because of its fixation with the lifestyles of the middle-class gentrifier rather than any serious attention being given to the working class and the displaced. Loïc Wacquant concurred, stating, 'any rigorous study of gentrification would seem *ex definitionis* to hold together the trajectories of the lower-class old timers and of the higher-class newcomers battling over the fate of the revamped district, since this class nexus forms the very heart of the phenomena' (Wacquant 2008: 199). Others have noted this tendency (e.g. Paton 2014) but precious few have subsequently paid much attention to the lives of the displaced, or offered a working-class perspective on gentrification. The question is why? One answer is the methodological: Tom Slater (2006) suggests careful qualitative consideration of working-class people and how gentrification affects them is lacking because of the difficulty of tracking the lives of the working classes and the displaced. But this emphasis on method is, argues Wacquant, less important than what he depicts as an almost ideological eviction of critical perspectives around gentrification and a 'class blindness' which mirrors the objectification of the working class over recent decades.

In this book, I have argued that policies for the revitalization of British High Streets have been accepted almost without question, to the extent few appear to be making the equation between retail regeneration and the displacement of the poorer in society. This is repeated in other national contexts, and even in the USA, where retail gentrification has been most debated, critical analyses sometimes appear somewhat ambivalent about retail change. Tom Slater (2006) highlights this when he notes that Sharon Zukin—perhaps the most influential interpreter of changing patterns of urban consumption—adopts an almost celebratory tone in some of her descriptions of the gentrification of East Village, New York, arguing in a co-authored piece that 'far from destroying a community by commercial gentrification, East Ninth Street suggests that a retail concentration of designer stores may be a territory of innovation in the urban economy, producing both a marketable and a sociable neighbourhood node' (Zukin and Kosta 2004: 101). Likewise, Phil Kasinitz and Sharon Zukin (2016: 55) argue that Orchard Street, also on the Lower East Side, has been 'successfully revitalized by new investment, restaurants and retail stores', shaking off its 'ghetto image' with no attendant 'crisis in moral ownership.' Here, there's little said about class conflicts, with the obvious onset of retail gentrification scripted as regenerative rather than necessarily driving a wedge between the poorer and the more affluent. Indeed, instead of focusing on class conflict on the High Street, much of the discussion in the USA seems to be about ethnicity, with the continuing presence of businesses being run by immigrants taken as evidence of a resilient retail 'ecosystem', irrespective of whom those businesses are catering for or what they are selling (see also Hentschel and Blokland 2016).

What seems to happening here is a collective amnesia about why we study gentrification: that is, to expose the processes which result in the displacement of working-class populations from the spaces where they live and work. Indeed, the subtitle of this section refers to a book probably little known beyond those working in queer activism, but highly pertinent in this context. Sarah Schulman's (2012) *The Gentrification of the Mind: witness to a lost imagination* is a slim but powerful book in which she makes connections between the consequences of AIDS, the literal gentrification of the city and a 'diminished consciousness' about how political and social change occurs. Her argument, though backed up by anecdote rather than empirical data, is powerfully persuasive, and relates to what she sees as the erasure of a 'queer urban ecology' due to the combined effects of deaths from HIV, in the first instance, and, secondly, the gentrification of New York. Here, she hypothesizes the injection of new middle-class money into previously mixed neighbourhoods—many of which were decimated by HIV and AIDS—created spaces more homogeneous in class terms than their predecessors. The eviction of the less affluent, she argued, reduced urbanity: white middle-class suburban cultural values came to reign where previously diverse ones had mingled and clashed. Yet, over time, she argues these gentrified neighbourhoods became normalized as made by the middle classes, with incomers forgetting these neighbourhoods had even existed before they 'created' them. As she sees it, the failure of the gentrifiers—many of them gay white men—to acknowledge the previous lower-class inhabitants of the area, including people of colour who had been active in the struggle against AIDS, is testament to 'the loss of a generation's ideas'. As Shulman states, gentrified happiness requires the gentrification of the mind, and the forgetting of what has been suffered—and achieved—by previous generations.

This argument, though specific to a particular queer struggle, has considerable resonance for my consideration of British High Streets. While I do not wish to assume we are all bourgeois now, the narrative surrounding the High Street is hardly contested at all. The idea that High Streets are dying, and that their revivification needs to involve the replacement of certain land uses, shops or facilities by more 'healthy' (read: wealthy) outlets, boutiques and restaurants, is one that has become accepted as axiomatic in policy circles. Few challenge the idea that shabby and part-vacant High Streets need to be regenerated, tooled for the consumer society of the twenty-first century and made more attractive to those to the middle classes who have largely abandoned them in favour of out of town and online retailing. And as we wander down the street of the idealized High Street, with its mixture of chic vintage shops, independently run hipster cafés, and pop-up galleries, perhaps we are also all fooled into thinking this represents true urbanity because it appears so bohemian, not bourgeois, and seems to signal cultural acceptance, diversity and opportunity. But, as I have stressed in this book, this diversity is only available to those who can afford it, and the gentrified High Street is far from accessible or open to all. The middle class, particularly its creative factions, imagine their access to food, art and culture on the High Street is due to their personal worth and hard work, yet their wealth is partly a function of their ability to define taste in favour of forms of cultural capital they are able to transform into economic capital. The gentrified High Street sets the standard for acceptability, normalizing the tastes and proclivities of the middle-class consumer in the process.

Schulmann (2012) argues gentrification is then the removal of the truly dynamic mix that defines urbanity, the privileging of a particular set of class dispositions and the disavowal of others. Despite claims to the contrary, the regeneration of the High Street predicated on this exact same logic: real social diversity and mix is shunned in favour of an upmarket form of consumption that feigns cosmopolitanism, looks good, and feels safe, but is palpably not for all (Fig. 10.1). But somehow this exclusionary logic has been forgotten. A gentrification of the mind has occurred. We still go to the High Street to experience urbanity, the juxtapositions of grit and glitter that have defined the urban condition, and taught us the importance of living alongside and encountering difference. But it's

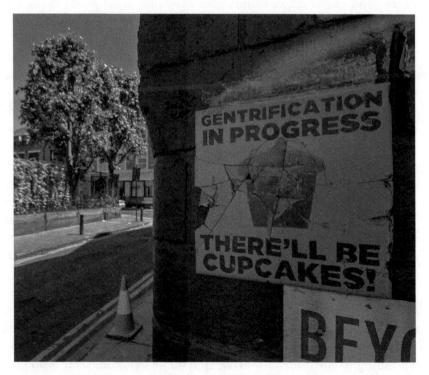

Fig. 10.1 The onset of gentrification, London, 2014 (photo: Sara Kelly, Flickr, used under a CCBY license)

apparent that, despite nods to the contrary, the contemporary, idealized High Street offers an *ersazt* urbanity not rooted in any particular time or place. And, for all the talk about creating High Streets that are not 'clone towns', tendencies towards homogenization are clearly evident, with the recipe for the successful High Street being rolled out the length and breadth of Britain.

The dominance of this model of High Street regeneration suggests the middle and upper classes have forgotten the lower classes have rights to the city too. In this sense, the gradual erasure of 'vulgar' working-class lives and lifestyles from the High Street helps us forget we live in societies where some people live precarious lives and where not all can take their allotted role as seduced consumers. At times, however, this illusion is punctured. Recall, for example, the English riots of 2011, which involved several nights of public disorder in the largest cities, manifest principally in the form of looting consumer goods from electrical goods shops and sportswear retailers. Although politicians were quick to denounce the riots as the work of 'feral' gangs (see Tyler 2013), and argued for a swift law and order response to quell an 'epidemic' of criminality, other commentators drew attention to the inequalities between those living in the poorer areas of cities and the growing affluence of the richest. Dan Dorling and Carl Lee (2014), for example, describe the disturbances as not merely symptomatic of a divided nation, but more specifically, of dividing cities. In their analysis they quote Ministry of Justice data to conclude 41% of those arrested for looting lived in the 10% of most deprived places in England, with 66% of those areas becoming poorer between 2007 and 2010. But more important, perhaps, was the fact many of these areas existed close to areas of affluent consumption. As Dorling and Lee highlight, where the poor remained relatively self-contained, and disconnected from wealthy areas or city centres, there was less evidence of rioting. Looting, it appears, is opportunistic, and few made extensive journeys to participate.

What this type of analysis suggests, as Owen Hatherley (2011) echoes, is that few of those involved in the riots lived in areas of concentrated poverty on the periphery or margins of the city: as he points out, in most British cities the poor live alongside, but oddly separate from, the rich, with this proximity often throwing up stark juxtapositions. He relates his own experience of living in London:

Occasionally, during the 12 years I've lived in the city, I'd often idly wonder when the riots would come: when the situation of organic delis next to pound shops, of crumbling maisonettes next to furiously speculated-on Victoriana, of artists shipped into architect-designed Brutalist towers to make them safe for regeneration, of endless boosterist self-congratulation, would finally collapse in on itself. (Hatherley 2011: np)

Hatherley expresses no surprise at the English riots, a moment when the 'socially excluded' decided they had had enough, would take what they wanted, 'what they couldn't afford and what they been told time and time again they were worthless without' (Hatherley 2011). Esteemed social theorist Zygmunt Bauman (2011) couches this somewhat differently, though his prognosis likewise asserts that the riots were the outcome of the toxic combination of spiralling consumerism and rising inequality. As he put it, 'this was not a rebellion or an uprising of famished and impoverished people or an oppressed ethnic or religious minority—but a mutiny of defective and disqualified consumers, people offended and humiliated by the display of riches to which they had been denied access… city riots in Britain are best understood as a revolt of frustrated consumers' (Bauman 2011: np). The implication here is that the parallel lives led by residents living in different areas of the city—some privileged, others associated with an 'underclass'—resulted in a moment of collapse when those living in deprived areas, often adjacent to areas of wealth, seized the consumer goods they felt they were denied by the accident of geography.

But if the future of the High Street is not as a gentrified, homogeneous space serving only the affluent, then what is it to be? Is it possible to imagine a diverse and resilient High Street that can reconcile the needs and tastes of different factions, or, as Bauman would have it, both the seduced and repressed? That very much depends on the extent to which these different factions are prepared to embrace the pleasures of being uncomfortable and are happy to mingle on local shopping streets, a process involving 'people with plural affiliations passing through, carrying multiple cares, sticking to familiar spaces, brushing past each other, bringing a host of pre-formed dispositions into the encounter' (Amin 2013: 62). It's hard to imagine this in a society where so much emphasis is put on the comfort and security of consumers and where many of the familiar tropes of urban management are about domestication through exclusion, not the fostering of everyday encounter. But one thing is for sure, and that is the gradual gentrification of a range of 'struggling' shopping spaces will leave a diminished range of retail options for the less affluent.

High Streets for the Poor

As we have seen, a key conceit informing current retail policy in Britain is that High Streets are dying, with the town centres of smaller urban settlements particularly vulnerable to the combined threat of online retail and out of town shopping. But if we pick at this discourse, it becomes apparent the death of the British High Street is much exaggerated. Certainly, some towns exhibit high vacancy rates, but in most instances is not proving so hard to re-let the properties 'abandoned' by the retail multiples to new businesses. For example, three years' after the demise of *Woolworths*, the Local Data Company (2012) pointed out that 87% of the 800 plus properties once occupied by this High Street chain had been re-let, the majority actually at higher rentals than before. In many senses, it's what they had been replaced by which appears to fuel the 'death' of the High Street thesis—pound shops, betting shops, discount stores and their ilk. These are all viable businesses, but their proliferation has been taken to indicate that some (perhaps many) High Streets are undergoing a series of transformations that amount to a 'downgrading'. But why is it a problem that High Streets are adapting by meeting the needs of poorer groups in times of recession? Do we really need to encourage gentrification as a way of 'reviving' them? In this book, I have argued current attempts at regeneration can hence be described as examples of revanchism—i.e. attempts by the middle classes to 'take back' the central city—tied into ongoing urban agendas oriented towards property speculation and gentrification.

Here, my own observations on the role of High Streets in promoting vernacular creativity, conviviality, and senses of belonging suggest that representations of incivility and abandonment do not tell the whole story of local shopping streets in Britain. Following Suzanne Hall (2012: 95) in particular, I conclude it's vital that High Streets remain 'shared local spaces shaped by habitual associations rather than outright compatibilities', being an 'aggregation of small spaces and diverse groups' that create 'local' cultures and senses of belonging (see also Amin 2010). In societies where there's much diversity, and both affluence and poverty, the High Street is never going to fulfill the same role for everyone, but we need to recapture the sense that there can be a variety of different users and uses present. To put this more straightforwardly, shops do not need to look, or function, like boutiques to play an important role on High Street. In my time in Margate, for example, I have come to see that betting shops, charity shops, and fast food restaurants all play valuable, although different, roles as spaces of sociality and consumption. So too do some of the corporate venues hipsters shun in their search for 'alternative' and authentic consumption. We should not underestimate the role chains like *Costa* or *Greggs* play as meeting places and the fact that people of different class and ethnic origin appear to be comfortable in using them. While they might be dismissed as serialized and inauthentic, they can serve as sites of what Hannah Jones et al. (2015) refer to as 'embedded localism'. Their study of franchised coffee shops as spaces of everyday encounter underlines this, suggesting:

> The familiarity and homogeneity of the cafés' layout, menus and expected practices make it possible for a range of uses to be projected onto them. They act in this way for people of multiple ethnicities, with multiple migratory histories, of different class and life course positions and across gender. The regularity and standardization of corporate cafés allow them to function as 'open' to confident use in a way that more boutique, specifically 'ethnic' or intensely 'local' consumption spaces may not. (Jones et al. 2015: 657)

This conclusion resonates strongly with my own observations, based on long afternoons in the *Costa* on Margate High Street watching the constant coming and going of different clientele, including long meetings of mother and baby groups, family reunions, child-minders handing over kids to their parents, business meetings, and so on. They alone read the free newspapers provided, and some plug their laptops in to surf the web. There's not much spontaneous mixing, but nor do there seem to be any awkward encounters. No-one ever looks particularly out of place, and dwelling is not discouraged. It's also relatively affordable. Not cheap, perhaps, but certainly cheaper than some of the more 'twee' cafés and cupcake shops in the gentrified Old Town.

But this focus on chain and franchised businesses should not overshadow the role some overtly 'ethnicised' businesses continue to play on many High Streets. Tim Townshend (2016) argues as much when he suggests the displacement of shopping by 'ethnic' food outlets has provided valuable meeting spaces in some communities, and also injected a sense of vitality in struggling areas. As Hall (2012) shows, these can also be important as spaces connecting local to global, with both owners and customers often engaged in something other than merely business. These may sometimes be marginalized outlets where the proprietor has to work long hours to make a living wage, but this does not necessarily mean they need to market themselves to knowing white cosmopolitan consumers, to play a useful economic as well as social role (see Kuppinger 2014). For example, the small, unnamed Polish-run Mini Market on Margate High Street is cluttered, and fairly expensive compared to the local supermarket, but it's open pretty much constantly, and offers an impressive range of imported Polish beers and tinned food alongside lottery tickets, milk, bread, cigarettes, and newspapers, a contemporary update of the traditional 'open all hours' corner shop that has always been an important presence on the High Street. Like the *Priceless* discount shop a few doors away, whose £1 sets of dusters, kitchen rolls and plastic washing up bowls spill haphazardly onto the pavement this could easily be dismissed as a transient business, a site of ad hoc retailing that has only a passing hold on the High Street (Fig. 10.2). But when I enquire in the latter, the woman behind the counter proudly tells me the shop was established 'about twenty-five years ago'. Far from being a short-lived 'pop-up', discount shops and those catering primarily to working-class shoppers can be long-term sustainable businesses, and it should not be assumed these represent a transient land use easily sacrificed in the name of retail regeneration (Hunt 2015). So while it's tempting to describe a High Street like Margate's as in a 'state of suspension', waiting for more permanent retail businesses to take root, this is to miss the point that it already serves local populations and does not need a regeneration involving the replacement of 'ethnic' or discount stores by boutiques, art galleries and cafés run by white hipsters.

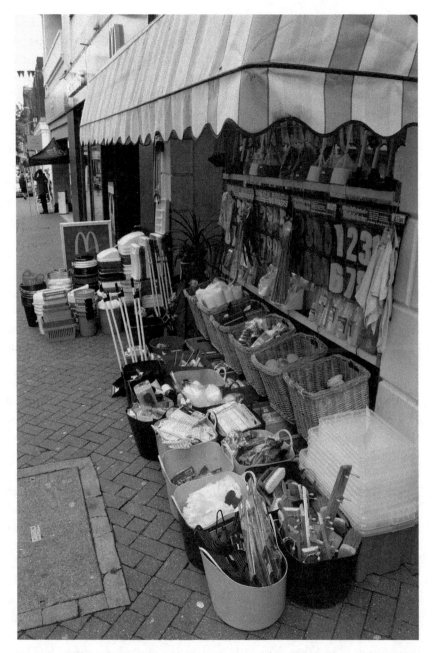

Fig. 10.2   Disordered but diverse? Priceless DIY store, Margate (photo: author)

Emphasizing the social, cultural and economic role of sometimes maligned businesses in this way is important given the contemporary regeneration rhetoric describing many High Streets as failing. In this rhetoric we see the repetition of discourses identifying some existing land uses and shops—e.g. fast food takeaways, betting shops, payday lenders, charity shops, lap dance clubs, bargain booze pubs—as easily sacrificed in the name of 'regeneration'. But, as we have seen, opposition to some of these is not really about their economic contribution to the High Street, being based instead on classed assumptions that these serve as a repository for unruly, debased and unmanageable identities. Others are seen as merely cheap, selling goods of questionable value that do not bequeath any distinction on those purchasing them. In this book, I have shown that a language of disgust is threaded through the opposition to such premises, betraying the fears projected onto the working classes by a popular media that represents them as vulgar, tasteless and dangerous (see also Haylett 2001). As such, I have argued the type of High Street envisaged in contemporary policy circles—where fried chicken gives way to cupcakes, and where customers sip craft beers rather than sip a pint of *Wetherspoons'* lager—is grounded in a set of classed assumptions about 'respectable' modes of behaviour and morality.

Such questions of value, morality and taste matter. They matter because, contrary to some characterizations of contemporary society, we are not all middle class. The simple fact is, that despite politicians' claims, Britain remains deeply divided, with many among the unemployed and working poor simply unable to consume in the manner which many of the dominant models of High Street seem to assume are 'normal'. The Portas Review, and some of the subsequent activities associated with the Portas Town Team, suggested a strategy based on creating a vibrant and attractive High Street built around food and arts culture, the cultivation of local heritage, the involvement of young people and community partnerships would 'save' Margate High Street. Here, no doubt, envious eyes were cast down the coast to towns like Whitstable, regularly identified as the town with the highest proportion of independent, local traders, and one which had developed a reputation for food and drink which is in keeping with its harbor-based and fishing heritage. Perhaps those involved in Margate's retail regeneration were also inspired by Deal, also on the Kent coast, voted High Street of the Year 2014 by readers of *The Daily Telegraph* in recognition of its distinctive mixture of retail chains (including some, like *Marks and Spencer*, that long ago abandoned Margate) as well as antique shops, vintage boutiques and 'real' coffee shops. But Margate's population is, on average, less affluent than that of Deal, and a good deal less wealthy than that of Whitstable.

Over the last couple of years there have been perceptible changes on Margate's High Street, particularly at the lower end where vintage shops, smart cafés and secondhand bookshops have sprung up, no doubt hoping to attract the 'Down from Londons' and Turner Contemporary visitors as they wander back to the train station. But whether this Portas-approved recipe for retail regeneration is the right way for its High Street to develop, needs to be questioned. The Old Town already offers boho-chic for the London hipsters, and whether the town really needs more cupcake shops or vintage boutiques is debatable. In reality, Margate High Street needs to be more than just a space designed to attract visitors to spend a few pounds a couple of times a year. The High Street is a thoroughfare for local people, a focus for social life, a space to sit and watch the world go by. It needs to be lively, engage different populations and of course cater to different tastes and pockets. Margate is not just for white middle-class incomers, artists and investors; it's also for those who have lived in the town for generations, as well as recent incomers from Europe and beyond. Most of the latter are not wealthy, and they have come to the town because its housing is comparatively cheap (at least when compared with London and much of the rest of Kent). Do these populations really want more barista coffee, burlesque-style vintage corsets and distressed coffee tables?

In raising such questions, I am not suggesting an empty shop is better than a shop targeted at the more affluent. But I am asking for a more open debate about the needs of local populations, and recognition of their tastes and lifestyles. Margate's population is massively different to the more affluent Whitstable, so why should it aspire to have the same kind of gentrified, twee High Street? Surely there are better role models elsewhere? Take the examples of the Walworth Road or Rye Lane in South London, two streets examined by Suzanne Hall. Few retail analysts seem to get excited about High Streets like these, but as Hall (2013: 1) argues, they 'exhibit a relative economic and cultural vibrancy despite being located within areas of relatively high deprivation'. These High Streets boast few empty shops, they are always busy, and the stores, many owned by first generation immigrants from North Africa, South East Asian and the Caribbean are important spaces of sociality for different groups. They are certainly not polished, in fact they are pretty rough and ready. But they are vibrant and vital, and serve the needs of local people pretty well with their variety of 'ethnic' food stores, chemists, convenience stores, phone shops as well as bookmakers, moneylenders, pubs, and chicken shops (something Carmona 2014, similarly argues in the case of Redbridge High Street). Some of these businesses fall well outside official visions of what the High Street should contain, but they create jobs, and offer affordable diversion and leisure, adding to the diversity and vibrancy of the High Street even if they are frowned on by the middle classes who consider premises like betting shops or fast food takeaways to be blighting our towns and cities.

So in the wake of The Portas Review, there's a lot of pressure to transform 'failing' High Streets into something quite different, and with this comes the danger of retail gentrification producing something, not for local populations at all. My hope is that future policies for the High Street recognize that although the number of shops on some local shopping streets may be declining, it's still a well-used space where people go to take out money, buy lottery tickets, search for bargains in charity shops, make convenience purchases, or simply sit and watch the world go by from a cheap pub or café. It's this type of 'unspectacular' and uncelebrated activity we need to nurture and develop if High Streets are to serve the needs of varied populations rather than just those of gentrifying incomers and tourists.

References

Amin, A. (2010). *Cities and the ethic of care for the stranger. Joint Joseph Rowntree Foundation/University of York Annual Lecture.* York: Joseph Rowntree Foundation.

Amin, A. (2013). *Land of Strangers.* Chichester: John Wiley.

Atkinson, R. (2003). Domestication by cappuccino or a revenge on urban space? Control and empowerment in the management of public spaces. *Urban Studies, 40*(9), 1829–1843.

Bauman, Z. (2011). Interview—Zygmunt Bauman on the UK riots. *Social Europe Journal*, Online Edition. Retrieved from www.social-europe.eu/2011/08/interview-zygmunt-bauman-on-the-uk-riots/

Carmona, M. (2014). London's local High Streets: The problems, potential and complexities of mixed street corridors. *Progress in Planning,100*, 1–84.

Coleman, R. (2004). Watching the degenerate: CCTV and urban regeneration. *Local Economy, 19*(3), 199–211.

Department of Communities and Local Government (DCLG) (2013). *The future of High Streets*. London: DCLG.

Dorling, D., & Lee, C. (2014). Inequality constitutes a particular place. In D. Pritchard & F. Pakes (Eds.), *Riot, unrest and protest on the global stage*. Palgrave Macmillan: Basingstoke.

Findlay, A., & Sparks, L. (2012). Far from the 'Magic of the Mall': Retail (change) in 'other places'. *Scottish Geographical Journal, 128*(1), 24–41.

Grimsey, B. (2013) *The Grimsey Review: An alternative future for the High Street*. Retrieved from www.vanishinghighstreet.com

Hall, S. M. (2011). High Street adaptations: Ethnicity, independent retail practices, and localism in London's urban margins. *Environment and Planning A, 43*(11), 2571–2588.

Hall, S. M. (2012). *City, street and citizen: The measure of the ordinary*. London: Routledge.

Hall, S. M. (2013). *Future of London's town centres: Submission to the London Assembly's Planning Committee*. London: LSE Cities.

Hatherley, O. (2011) Looking at England's urban spaces, the riots were inevitable, https://www.opendemocracy.net/ourkingdom/owen-hatherley/look-at-englands-urban-spaces-riots-were-inevitable 17 August.

Haylett, C. (2001). Illegitimate subjects? Abject whites, neoliberal modernisation and middle class multiculturalism. *Environment and Planning D: Society and Space., 19*(3), 351–370.

Hentschel, C., & Blokland, T. (2016). Life and death of the great regeneration vision: Diversity, decay, and upgrading in Berlin's ordinary shopping streets. In S. Zukin, P. Kasinitz, & X. Chen (Eds.), *Global cities, local streets*. New York: Routledge.

High Street London (2010). *High Street London*. London: GLA.

Hubbard, P. (2006). *Key ideas in Geography—The City*. London: Routledge.

Hunt, M. (2015). Keeping shop, shaping place: The vernacular curation of London's *ad hoc* consumption spaces. PhD, Royal Holloway, University of London.

Jones, H., Neal, S., Mohan, G., Connell, K., Cochrane, A., & Bennett, K. (2015). Urban multiculture and everyday encounters in semi-public, franchised café spaces. *The Sociological Review, 63*(44), 644–661.

Kasinitz, P., & Zukin, S. (2016). From ghetto to global: Two neighbourhood shopping streets in New York City. In S. Zukin, P. Kasinitz, & X. Chen (Eds.), *Global cities, local streets*. New York: Routledge.

Kuppinger, P. (2014). A neighborhood shopping street and the making of urban cultures and economies in Germany. *City & Community, 13*(2), 140–157.

Lefebvre, H. (1991). *The production of space*. Oxford: Blackwell.

Local Data Company. (2012). *H2 vacancy rate report*. London: Local Data Company.

Paton, K. (2014). *Gentrification: A working class perspective*. Farnham: Ashgate.

Portas, M. (2011). The Portas review: An independent review into the future of our High Streets. http://www.maryportas.com/news/2011/12/12/the-portas-review/

Ravenscroft, N. (2000). The vitality and viability of town centres. *Urban Studies, 37*(13), 2533–2549.

Schulman, S. (2012). *The gentrification of the mind: Witness to a lost imagination*. Berkeley: University of California Press.

Shields, R. (1991). *Places on the margin*. London: Routledge.

Skeggs, B. (2009). The moral economy of person production: The class relations of self-performance on 'reality' TV. *The Sociological Review, 57*(4), 626–644.

Slater, T. (2006). The eviction of critical perspectives from gentrification research. *International Journal of Urban and Regional Research, 30*(4), 737–757.

Townshend, T. G. (2016). Toxic High Streets. *Journal of Urban Design*, online early, doi:10.1080/13574809.2015.1106916

Tyler, I. (2013). The riots of the underclass? Stigmatisation, mediation and the government of poverty and disadvantage in neoliberal Britain. *Sociological Research Online, 18*(4), 6.

Wacquant, L. (2008). Relocating gentrification: The working class, science and the state in recent urban research. *International Journal of Urban and Regional Research, 32*(1), 198–205.

Wrigley, N., & Dolega, L. (2011). Resilience, fragility and adaptation: New evidence on the performance of UK High Streets during global economic crisis and its policy implications. *Environment and Planning A, 43*(10), 2337–2363.

Zukin, S., & Kosta, E. (2004). Bourdieu off-Broadway: Managing distinction on a shopping block in the East Village. *City & Community, 3*(2), 101–114.

Index

© The Editor(s) (if applicable) and The Author(s) 2017
P. Hubbard, *The Battle for the High Street*,
DOI 10.1057/978-1-137-52153-8